INDIVIDUAL AND GROUP
COUNSELING IN SCHOOLS

The Guilford School Practitioner Series

EDITORS

STEPHEN N. ELLIOTT, Ph.D.
University of Wisconsin—Madison

JOSEPH C. WITT, Ph.D.
Louisiana State University, Baton Rouge

Academic Skills Problems: Direct Assessment and Intervention
EDWARD S. SHAPIRO

Curriculum-Based Measurement: Assessing Special Children
MARK R. SHINN (ED.)

Suicide Intervention in the Schools
SCOTT POLAND

Problems in Written Expression: Assessment and Remediation
SHARON BRADLEY-JOHNSON AND JUDI LUCAS LESIAK

Individual and Group Counseling in Schools
STEWART EHLY AND RICHARD DUSTIN

INDIVIDUAL AND GROUP COUNSELING IN SCHOOLS

STEWART EHLY, Ph.D.
RICHARD DUSTIN, Ph.D.
The University of Iowa

Foreword by Rickey L. George, Ph.D.

THE GUILFORD PRESS
New York   **London**

To Pam and Pat, for their continuing support.

© 1989 The Guilford Press
A Division of Guilford Publications, Inc.
72 Spring Street, New York, NY 10012

Printed in the United States of America

This book is printed on acid-free paper.

Last digit is print number: 9   8   7   6   5   4   3   2   1

Library of Congress Cataloging-in-Publication Data

Ehly, Stewart W., 1949–
    Individual and group counseling in schools / Stewart Ehly and Richard Dustin
      p. cm. — (The Guilford school practitioner series)
    Bibliography: p.
    Includes index.
    ISBN 0-89862-355-3. — ISBN 0-89862-234-4 (pbk.)
    1. Personnel service in education—United States. 2. Students—
Counseling of—United States. 3. Group guidance in education.
I. Dustin, E. Richard, 1936–   . II. Title.   III. Series.
    [DNLM: 1. Counseling—in adolescence. 2. Counseling—in infancy &
childhood. 3. Psychology, Educational. LB 1027.5 E33i]
LB1027.5.E355 1989
371.4—dc20
DNLM/DLC
for Library of Congress   89-11618
                                           CIP

Foreword

During the past two decades, there has been a marked increase in the number of counselors who work in a variety of nonschool settings. As a result, more and more counselor education programs and counseling textbooks have placed a primary emphasis on mental health settings outside the schools, leading to a decline in the literature written expressly for school counselors and which provides information on the unique problems that face individuals who offer counseling services within the schools.

Ehly and Dustin have rectified this situation. With only a brief overview of theories and strategies of counseling that have a general impact on all counseling, they highlight the ideas and concepts in terms of their specific application to schools and the uniqueness of the school setting. There seems to be little emphasis on theory itself, yet the ideas that are developed clearly are based solidly on theory. If one is looking for a thorough explanation of a particular theory, it is not here. But if one wishes to understand the application of that theory to the situation of the school counselor, this book will provide that understanding.

There are a number of features that are particularly impressive. The wealth of practical examples and the large number of exercises designed to provide an opportunity to practice a particular skill or strategy immediately are very unusual. My personal experience has been that coming up with such specific, meaningful exercises is much more difficult than writing the text itself. In addition, the book's numerous information boxes highlight and summarize the most important ideas presented. Going through and reading only the boxes would make the book highly worthwhile, even without reading the text. Of course, to do so would result in the reader failing to experience the value of the many practical examples and the clear description of the subtleties of those major points.

Ehly and Dustin also are unique in their separation of a major counseling service from the issues involved in providing that service in schools. The overview chapter on individual counseling in schools is followed by one that points out the practical issues involved in providing this service and then analyzes how the school counselor can best do so. The same process is found in their treatment of group counseling in schools. Even more worthwhile is their chapter on the practical issues related to school counseling in general, which is presented prior to the chapters on individual and group counseling and thus provides a perceptual framework for the rest of the book.

I can recall few instances where writers of a book designed to be a practical application of counseling services have placed such an emphasis on the evaluation of the effectiveness of those services. My experience has been that books focusing on theory and research almost always do so, but that because the emphasis on evaluation is somewhat separated from the practical in their minds, few counselors systematically evaluate what they do. Here the authors include evaluation as a practical issue and provide clear-cut guidelines on how to engage in evaluation with only minimal interference with the providing of counseling services.

The authors conclude with an analysis of the ethical and legal issues in counseling as they apply to the school setting. Their focus is on clear-cut examples of issues that exist in schools today, with strategies suggested for helping guide the school counselor toward ethically and legally appropriate behavior.

The practicality of this book suggests that the authors are closely allied with individuals who are school counselors today—individuals who want ideas and helpful suggestions to implement the theories they previously learned. The book certainly does not read like an edited transcript of a workshop, but has the best features of such a volume: clearly explained, practical ideas for the working professional school counselor.

I not only like this book, but am quite enthusiastic about it. Although I have been in the field since 1965, I learned a great deal from reading it. It is clear and basic enough for the new counselor and yet possesses the depth and practicality for the experienced counselor as well. I recommend *Individual and Group Counseling in Schools* for students of counseling, as well as for teachers, administrators, school social workers, and counselors who are in the field and who continue to search for ways to improve the work they do.

Rickey L. George, Ph.D.

Preface

The idea of counseling students is by no means a recent one, and an examination of the literature would verify how widely the topic has been addressed. Yet, too often, professionals and consumers fail to distinguish between the skills involved in counseling and the job title of "counselor." Many service providers in schools function in a counseling role on occasion, and some on a regular basis. The present text starts with the premise that, independent of the job title of the professional using such skills, the elements of effective counseling can be identified.

Professionals who practice in schools (called school practitioners in this text, and including teachers, administrators, counselors, and support personnel such as consultants, school psychologists, social workers, and so on) are often comfortable in talking with students, advising them on personal and school-related issues, yet would not claim to be practicing counseling. As we explore in the following chapters, discomfort at calling oneself a counselor, perhaps the best policy in an educational system that places a premium on certification standards, does not imply engaging in less than "best practices" when working with students. All school practitioners concerned with helping students deal with issues in their lives recognize an obligation to professional service at the highest standard of practice.

Thus, readers of this text will recognize a consistent theme throughout the chapters. All school practitioners who counsel students can enhance their abilities in the counseling role. Each professional can be a caring and influential individual prepared to attend to the needs of all students. We do not envision a school in which every staff member is a miniature counselor; rather, the contents of the text have been developed so that the school practitioner can understand what is involved in successful counseling and the consequences of agreeing to work with students on an individual or small group basis. We present an additional option, that of referring students for services, so that the reader can consider an alternative means of directing attention to children's needs.

The present text is written for all school practitioners interested in the elements of effective counseling. Students training for any of the roles found in the typical school will benefit from the materials by being introduced to the skills necessary for success in counseling-related encounters with children and adolescents. The text will alert students and professionals to the limits inherent to individual and small group counseling and will direct readers to resources containing additional information on theory and practice.

Finally, we promote a standard of ethical practice that involves the professional in ongoing reflection and monitoring of behavior. Too many of the professions that serve schools have not addressed dilemmas that confront practitioners in their daily work with children, parents, and colleagues. In the absence of a universal code of ethical behavior for school practitioners, we identify strategies that increase the likelihood of consistent attention to ethical practice.

Both authors would like to thank the series editors for their assistance throughout the writing of the manuscript. The useful feedback and words of encouragement were always helpful.

Contents

Chapter 1   Introduction   1
　Self Theory   3
　Adlerian Approaches   4
　Behavioral Approaches   6
　Cognitive Behavioral Approaches   7
　Who Practices Counseling in the Schools?   10
　Overview of This Book   12

Chapter 2   Issues Affecting Counseling   14
　Referral Considerations   14
　Counseling as a Direct or Indirect Service   18
　Counseling versus Consulting   19
　Barriers and Assets to Counseling   22
　Skills Contributing to Successful Counseling   25

Chapter 3   Individual Counseling   30
　Problems Addressed by Counseling   31
　Goals of Counseling   34
　Steps in the Counseling Process   39
　Identification of Students for Individual
　　Counseling   45
　Practical Implementation Issues   47
　Addendum: Skills for Interviewers   48

Chapter 4   Practical Issues of Individual Counseling   59
　Session-by-Session Points   59
　Useful Techniques for Individual Counseling   78
　Common Strategies for Dealing with Student Problems   84
　Conclusions   86

Chapter 5 Group Counseling   88
   Goals of Group Counseling 89
   Usefulness of Group Counseling 98
   Steps to Success in Group Counseling 100
   Summary 107

Chapter 6 Group Counseling: Process and Content   109
   Group Counseling Process 109
   Process Skills by Leaders 112
   Practical Leader Techniques 116
   Involving Students in Processing 122
   The Content of Group Counseling 123
   Content Common to Many Groups 126

Chapter 7 Evaluating the Effectiveness of Counseling   129
   The Process and Products of Counseling 129
   Looking at Products of Counseling 135
   Research and Counseling Outcomes 143
   Issues in Evaluating a Program of Counseling 145

Chapter 8 Ethical and Legal Issues   149
   Ethical Dilemmas 149
   Codes of Ethics 150
   Legal Dimensions of Service 155
   Legal Issues in Counseling 156
   Strategies to Enhance Ethical and Legal
     Decision Making 161

Appendix A Theoretical Influences on Counseling   166

Appendix B Further Readings   173

References   175

Index   179

1

Introduction

Counseling services are an important component of a school's offer-ings available to students and their parents. Counselors are just one of the many professionals who provide services that fall under the label of counseling. School psychologists, social workers, teachers, and even administrators engage in forms of counseling as part of their pro-fessional responsibilities. This book is intended to provide a brief introduction to counseling within the schools, alerting professionals to important dimensions of the strategies available to serve students in individual and group settings.

Counseling has been defined variously by a number of authors. Warner (1980), for example, defines counseling as

> a therapeutic and growth process through which individuals are helped to define goals, make decisions, and solve problems related to personal–social, educational and career concerns. Specialized counseling provides assistance with concerns related to physical and social rehabilitation, employment, mental health, substance abuse, marital and family prob-lems, human sexuality, religious and value choices, career development, and other concerns. (p. 2)

George and Cristiani (1986) have listed elements common to a number of the available definitions of counseling. The first is that counseling functions to assist people to make and act on choices. The second element of such definitions is that learning will occur as the result of counselor–client interactions. Such learning can be specific to the actions, thoughts, or emotions of the client or to some combina-tion thereof. A third element relates to personality development, although just what is meant by this notion differs across definitions. Essentially, with counseling, students can begin to understand better the dimensions of their personality and make decisions about changes that they can implement in their lives.

1

Although many school practitioners consider counseling a part of their job responsibilities, there are differences among professionals in the ways that they work with students. A teacher, for example, has little time (or training) to engage in extended individual counseling but may feel committed to working with the occasional student in need of personal attention and guidance. Similarly, a school psychologist may have the training to counsel students but spend the majority of his/her time conducting assessments and behavioral interventions. Another psychologist or school social worker, assigned to another setting, might spend half of each work day in counseling students. Preferences for service options as well as the needs and demands of the particular school will influence the professional's practice of counseling. We will consider differences among professionals and schools in the use of counseling interventions.

Most authors make an important distinction between counseling and psychotherapy (see Box 1.1). Counseling is generally seen, especially in school settings, as a relatively low-intensity intervention. Counseling consists of strategies that take place within a school setting rather than in a clinical or medical facility. Students who receive counseling are not considered to be mentally ill or functioning psychologically in a poor fashion. A student is not seen as a patient in the medical sense of the word, nor does the counselor work over as extensive a period of time as is typical in private practice settings. Most opportunities for counseling within the school setting are, almost by definition, brief in terms of available time and energies. Psychotherapy, in contrast, is an extended process that makes the assumption of poor psychological functioning on the part of the client. The role of the therapist allows for greater intensity of service as well as a larger commitment from clients.

BOX 1.1. Is It Counseling?

Educators, whether administrators, social workers, psychologists, or teachers, will frequently spend time with certain students either in groups or, more often, individually. The following is meant to suggest when these "get togethers" may qualify as counseling.

How to decide if student contacts are counseling-related:

1. Are you meeting more than twice?
2. Does the student ask for or seem to want the contact?
3. Are the purposes of the meetings agreed on by *both* the educator and the student?
4. Is there some noticeable progress toward these purposes?
5. Does the educator frequently listen and encourage the student to talk?

Counseling has been addressed from a number of theoretical perspectives (see Box 1.2). Some of these perspectives will be important for this text in that we will focus discussion on the most widely used approaches to service. Considered briefly at this time will be Adlerian, Rogerian, behavioral, and cognitive approaches to counseling. These four approaches were selected because of their influential role within the development of educational counseling and because of the ease with which certain theoretical principles and techniques can be applied to limited counseling within an educational setting. This discussion is not intended to denigrate the importance of other theoretical perspectives, especially since the influence of these approaches is evident in services offered by professional counselors in schools.

SELF THEORY

Carl Rogers has had a profound effect on the entire field of counseling in both clinical and school settings. His ideas developed within the context of client-centered therapy have been widely applied with children and adults. In fact, during the 1950s and '60s, no other system had such widespread impact in vocational counseling, Veterans Administration hospitals, schools, and employment settings. Important components of Rogers's ideas about services include constructs of positive regard for others, self-regard, conditions of worth, conditions of normal development, and problems in living. His exten-

---

BOX 1.2. Handout: Usefulness of a Theory—Personal Checklist

The reader is urged to apply each item in the following list to each of the four approaches to counseling that follow. The intent is to clarify your understanding of each system and also to focus your values and beliefs toward aspects of each system that may be attractive and practical for you.

1. Is the theory understandable to me? Do I find the key terms and constructs sensible?
2. Each of the approaches focuses on elements of the human condition (feelings for Rogers, cognitions for Ellis and other cognitive writers, etc.). Do the students with whom I spend time or wish to spend time have problems and needs that go along with this system?
3. Do the goals of this system seem useful to me in light of the above (2)?
4. Can I see myself practicing the essential techniques of this theory? Note: Chapters 3 through 6 contain the useful techniques for counseling in educational settings. Perhaps it is too early to reach a conclusion.
5. Does the theory suggest a method of evaluation? How can I tell when I've helped a student? When do I need to get some help?
6. Other.

---

sive writings on the development of children include an emphasis on
the positive, a focus he maintains throughout the entire course of the
counseling process. For example, an important assumption about
people according to Rogerian counselors is that only the individual
student can know what course of action is "right" for him/her. In
other words, each person possesses the essential characteristics to
become the optimal person possible. The Rogerian counselor has
been described as providing the essential ingredients that allow a
student to "blossom." These ingredients are delivered by the counsel-
or within a special relationship that is the essential component of
Rogerian counseling.

During counseling, Rogers emphasizes maintaining minimum anxi-
ety for the client as activities are attempted to help bring about
problem resolution. The counselor should communicate in a fashion
that enhances genuineness, unconditional positive regard, empathic
understanding, and accurate client perception. The client's worth
must be maintained and enhanced through all components of the
counseling process. Rogers was much less concerned with counseling
techniques than with enacting a sense of presence that would allow
the client to explore himself/herself and to grow psychologically.

More recent writing by Carkhuff (1973) and Gazda (1973) has
expanded on many of Rogers's ideas. In Chapter 3 of this text, an
extended discussion is provided of the communication skills that
Rogers considered essential for successful counseling. The more recent authors have attempted to operationalize certain constructs of
Rogerian counseling, especially the techniques. For example, *empathy*
has become "reflection of feelings," wherein the counselor communicates an understanding of the feeling just expressed by the
client. *Unconditional positive regard* has become "genuineness," wherein
the counselor communicates so that his/her nonverbal communication does not conflict or detract from the content or verbal communication. Although many writers have recently "translated" Rogerian counseling into more specific terms and techniques, the lack of
emphasis on "action" or specific behavioral change has reduced the
popularity of this system for counselors within an educational setting.

ADLERIAN APPROACHES

Alfred Adler, in breaking away from previous psychoanalytic tradi-
tions and therapy techniques, developed and applied concepts of
helping others that have been integrated into many counseling
approaches. Much of Adler's conceptual development was conducted

with parents and staff of educational institutions around the turn of the 20th century. Adler believed that human beings are motivated primarily by a sense of social responsibility and a need to achieve. His priorities for the human being were much more humanistic than Freud's ideas based on sexual and aggressive drives. For Adler, individuals are pulled by goals that are partially of their own choosing and are not necessarily under the absolute control of their unconscious.

Adler perceived human beings as striving toward what he called a life's goal. Such goals revolve around that person's perceptions of the environment, which were influenced by family structure, parental actions, and sibling interactions. Interestingly, Adlerian counselors would accept the client's *report* of the family structure or the actions of the parent. In this regard, Rogerian and Adlerian counselors would *not* concern themselves with corroborating the stories of a student but would work from the perspective of the client.

Adler developed the notion of *life-style*, although for him the ideas had little to do with our modern day conceptions of this term. Lifestyle centered around the idea that individuals develop a pattern of interacting with the environment based on inner perceptions of the environment as well as past successes and failures relating to others, especially members of the immediate family. Adler also saw the individual as developing within a social environment that resulted in what he labeled "social interest." Children who had problems in school were often considered to have failed in important aspects of their development of social interest and life-style. Their problems could be seen as mistaken goals of behavior. Important goals of misbehavior include a desire for attention, a desire for power, an urge for retaliation, and a belief of helplessness.

Much of what Adler discussed in terms of counseling did not include an emphasis on techniques of the counselor. Adler's followers, such as Dreikurs (see, for example, Dreikurs & Soltz, 1964) and Dinkmeyer (see, for example, Dinkmeyer & Carlson, 1973), have been instrumental in proposing techniques based on Adler's theoretical concepts.

The process of Adlerian counseling involves understanding the client's life-style as well as the circumstances of its development. Techniques include empathy, intuition, and interpretation and center on understanding patterns of behavior exhibited by the client. By understanding behavior and others' reaction to it, the counselor is able to interpret life-style and provide direction for the student and that child's teachers and parents so that more positive behaviors can be developed. In addition, it is important to an Adlerian counselor that the child/client also gains an understanding of his/her own behavior. Adler's notions of encouragement, logical consequences, and democratic practices have played an important part in counseling and education, as will be described in upcoming chapters on counseling approaches. Professional groups, usually called individual psychology (IP) groups, exist in all parts of the United States and offer an interested educator a fascinating opportunity to learn about and to become more involved in Adlerian concepts and educational ideas.

BEHAVIORAL APPROACHES

Behavioral counseling has developed from earlier experimental activities with animals and human beings, much of which was stimulated by the work of B. F. Skinner. Notions such as reinforcement, extinction, generalization, discrimination, and shaping have entered the vocabulary of educators and support professionals interested in bringing about changes in student behaviors. The broader notion of learning theory has provided the philosophical and theoretical basis for much of what occurs in behavioral approaches. Counselors using the behavioral approach will not assume that a child is bad or good but rather will work to understand how the child's environment supports certain behaviors that others consider to be improper or problematic. This practice follows directly from the view of humans as *tabula rasa*. Humans are neither good nor bad but are capable of learning any type of behavior.

By understanding the conditions under which behavior occurs, the counselor can work to make modifications in client actions. The environment, rather than the student, holds the "controls" for behaviors. Such concerns as what immediately precedes the behavior and what conditions that follow the behavior may be serving to reinforce it are examples of factors important to a behavioral counselor. Goals of counseling using the behavioral approach include achieving problem definition in concrete language, acquiring a developmental and social history, establishing specific goals of counseling, and determining methods to bring about desired change (Hansen, Stevic, & Warner, 1982). The goals for behavioral counseling might be to increase a desired behavior, to decrease a dysfunctional behavior, or to develop strategies for combining both.

Techniques of counseling involve contracting for change, behavioral shaping, systematic desensitization, and related practices of modeling and reinforcement of incompatible behaviors. There are many different approaches to behavioral counseling; thus, practitioners can be extremely diverse in what they practice. However, it is important to underscore the nature of behavioral *counseling*. As indicated in Box 1.1, counseling includes the optional involvement of the student. This aspect of the voluntariness of behavioral counseling, more than any other single criterion, separates it from such other behavioral practices as behavior modification or behavioral therapy.

COGNITIVE BEHAVIORAL APPROACHES

A more recent approach than the previous three involves the work of writers such as Albert Ellis (1973), Maxie Maultsby (1975), and many others. This approach developed in response to criticisms leveled at behavioral notions, arguing that humans are more than a tally of behaviors, that humans also possess thoughts, hopes, aspirations, and dreams. Currently the most popular approach to counseling is the cognitive approach. Researchers have attested to lasting changes with clients (instead of short-term gains) by applying the principles of learning to the thoughts and language patterns of clients.

Ellis (1962) developed the approach to counseling called "rational emotive theory" (RET), and Maultsby (1975) is better known for his work on "rational behavioral therapy" (RBT). Both authors stress that many of the problems that children as well as adults experience are based on what they label faulty beliefs. Thoughts that individuals have as they consider actions play an important role in eventual interactions with others and the emotions related to those interactions (see Box 1.3).

A counselor using an RET or RBT approach will work to influence illogical thoughts. As described in Box 1.4, counselors using Ellis's approach believe that thinking causes feelings. In those cases in which the feelings of clients are disruptive to their lives, and when symptoms exist such as lateness of assignments, absenteeism, or bullying, then the counselor would predict irrational (*B* in Box 1.3) rather than rational thought. Illogical thoughts are best identified with the cooperation of the client. Box 1.4 describes how one educator worked on the illogical thoughts of a student.

A variety of techniques are available from Ellis and Maultsby to use with students. Both authors borrow strategies used by behaviorists, Adlerian psychologists, and Rogerian counselors, recognizing the effectiveness of related theoretical orientations. Although little of this textbook is devoted to RET and RBT approaches, Appendix B contains references on many important resources for applying

BOX 1.3. The ABC's of Ellis's Counseling

A: Activating event
B: Self-talk
C: Feelings

Activating events—having to stay after school, being assigned detention—don't cause feelings. The individual's thoughts do. Therefore, it is "irrational" according to rational emotive counseling to say, "That teacher makes me so mad."

However, not all feelings require counseling, nor are they prerequisites for receiving help. The practitioner using this system would start by listening and using the communication skills that help lead to trust and honest expression. These techniques are described in Chapters 3 and 4.

When the student/client states that the feelings are disruptive—interfering with goals, causing undesirable consequences—the counselor teaches the clients the ABC's. For example, "You say that these feelings of sadness about breaking up with your boyfriend have lasted too long and that you want to let them go. Well, I think your boyfriend didn't cause your sad feelings, but that you must be telling yourself something *about* his breaking up with you. Is that possible?"

No matter how the student responds, sometimes it is necessary to repeat yourself; then, the counselor obtains commitment from the client.

For example, "I know it isn't really clear just yet, but are you willing to help me see if we can discover what you may be telling yourself about the break-up? See, I think everyone does this—that we cause our own difficulties. Will you help me try?"

If no commitment can be obtained, then this type of counseling, and perhaps any type, is not recommended.

Now, when irrational thoughts are causing misery, Ellis suggests D and E to follow the ABC's.

A: My boyfriend doesn't like me anymore.
B: Irrational message. For example: "He shouldn't treat me this way." "He has no right to break up with me." "I'll never be in love again."
C: The miserable, disruptive feeling.
D: Counselor *disputes*—only the irrational thought. "*Should* has nothing to do with it. You say he did dump you. You say he won't speak to you and that he's flirting with someone else. There is no *should* here. It may be embarrassing; it may be uncomfortable, but it isn't *awful*. In fact, you can stand it. You have stood it this long, and at times with me, you have even laughed and had your old spark."

The counselor continues to dispute—hammer—argue, but only with the irrational thought, until the two can substitute a more rational thought.

E: Act out appropriate behavior. Client shows that he/she can recognize his/her own irrational thoughts—no one escapes from them—not even educators—but many of us can learn to recognize them and how we are making ourselves miserable.

BOX 1.4. Counseling an Adolescent

Although, the following example is a very mild case, it illustrates the steps that were described in Box 1.3.

Jerry reported that he hadn't done his homework because of his friends. Since he was very busy, Mr. E had Jerry come in during study hall.

Mr. E: Now, tell me again, Jerry, how your friends didn't let you do your homework.

J: Well, that's right. They all wanted to go to the mall, so I didn't have a chance to do it. [**A:** Activating event]

Mr. E: It would help me, Jerry, if I know how you felt. Your friends wouldn't let you do the assignment. How do you feel about it?

J: I don't know. I guess I'm mad at them. [**C:** Feelings]

Mr. E: You know I don't think your friends are the reason you didn't do the homework. It was your responsibility. Even though you wanted to go to the mall, you didn't have to. [**D:** Disputing]

J: You don't know them. They really have fun. They wanted me to go.

Mr. E: But you knew you had homework. You chose to go. Then instead of taking responsibility for your choice, you blamed them. You used them for an excuse. Isn't that right?

J: I guess so.

Mr. E: Now, so you need the points from the homework?

J: I guess so.

Mr. E: Do you or not? Do you understand the grading system?

J: Yes. I want a B, and I do need the homework points.

Mr. E: So next time, when you have homework, what might you do?

J: What do you mean?

Mr. E: Jerry, come on. You know what I mean. There is homework due tomorrow. If your friends want to do something, what can you do?

J: I guess I can tell them I have homework.

Mr. E: It might not be fun; it might not even be what you would like to do; but you're right. You could say, "I can't guys, I have homework." Now what should I expect from you when tomorrow's assignment is due?

Here Mr. E is getting commitment from Jerry. Commitment and contractual agreements are often used with cognitive systems.

---

these approaches in school counseling. Additional sources of information on theories discussed above appear in Appendix A.

Some rational emotive counselors are seen as aggressive and argumentative in their work with clients. Indeed, such counselors do utilize techniques that force the client to confront thoughts, beliefs, and feelings. Although it may not be apparent to a casual observer, the counselor is attacking *only* the illogical thought of the client, not the client. One of us once asked a school counselor about the purpose of his shouting at a student, and the counselor explained, "Oh, I use rational emotive counseling." However, as the excerpt in Box 1.5 shows, the counselor communicates many of the caring and understanding tendencies of an Adlerian or Rogerian counselor while helping the client discover just what irrational thoughts are causing the disruptive feelings. Box 1.5 indicates one author's rules for what constitutes "rational thought."

WHO PRACTICES COUNSELING IN THE SCHOOLS?

Counseling has been described as one of the preferred methods of intervention with immature and unmanageable students (Algozzine, Ysseldyke, Christenson, & Thurlow, 1982). In addition, sometimes the lost and lonely student is a prime candidate for special time and the undivided attention of the educator. Counseling can be seen as one of many alternative services for psychoeducational intervention. For those practitioners who can identify many students who seem to demand excessive amounts of attention and time, counseling offers an alternative whereby the student *earns* the time with the teacher. As Box 1.1 indicates, counseling requires progress, a focus, and a sense of accomplishment; whenever students don't seem to be making such progress, the need for counseling may be ended. Terminating and referring clients will be discussed later, especially in Chapter 2.

Because counseling in schools focuses on current and future problem solving of students who are relatively able to cope, a number of people in the schools can engage in counseling interventions. By role definition, school counselors are important components of a total service program involving counseling. School psychologists have re-

---

BOX 1.5. Rules for Rational Behavior

Physical and emotional behavior is rational if it obeys at least three of these five rules.

1. Behavior is based on objective reality or the known relevant facts of a situation.
2. Behavior enables you to protect your life.
3. Behavior enables you to achieve your goals most quickly.
4. Behavior enables you to keep out of significant trouble with other people.
5. Behavior enables you to prevent or quickly eliminate significant personal emotional conflict.

Source: Adapted from Maultsby, M. C., Jr. (1975). *Help yourself to happiness through rational self-counseling.* Boston: Marlborough House.

cently begun to engage in much more counseling, primarily at a secondary school level. Social workers, classroom teachers, and administrators may opt to be involved in limited counseling within the normal range of their activities. All too often, practitioners who are effective listeners or skilled counselors find many students absorbing large amounts of their time, but with no clear result. The four types of counseling presented in this text emphasize a purpose and a focus in counseling. Services delivered under the label of "counseling" will differ from simple advice giving or "shoulder to cry on" support that any nontrained person can apply with students. The ideas for counseling, as presented in this text, will assist school practitioners to identify useful techniques for doing more than being a passive listener to students' problems. We will promote the notion that counseling conducted by noncounselors be limited in intent to match the student's needs and the professional's skills.

Changes in the way that services are delivered in schools will play an important part in the future of counseling within school settings. Some states are combining the roles of support service professionals so now there are no longer individual psychologists, counselors, and social workers but rather a more generically labeled mental health service provider made available to students and parents. In other schools, entire job classifications have been removed for economic reasons. Some districts, for example, have lost elementary school counselors because the districts could not support counseling services at that grade level. At the same time, one state (Iowa) has recently mandated that all school districts have elementary counselors. As services are eliminated and redefined, practitioners in any setting must examine priorities for service and available resources for delivering counseling to students and parents.

A study by Dustin, Ehly, and Curran (1984) noted that counselors and psychologists placed a high priority on counseling at all grade levels as a service of choice. Regardless of the professionals' theoretical orientations, counseling was considered to be a very important segment of the total package of psychoeducational services delivered.

One difficulty in some school districts is that too few professionals are providing effective group and individual counseling relative to student needs. In those districts, school practitioners can elect to play an important role in helping students through counseling, especially when full-time providers of counseling services are not meeting needs.

Parents are generally very supportive of counseling, especially when it is combined with guidance services. Unfortunately, little empirical evidence has been generated in support of counseling interventions with students. Research that has compared counseling to teacher consultation or behavior management of the students has concluded that both of these approaches are more effective in producing behavior change than is counseling (Marlowe, Madsen, Bowen, Reardon, & Logue, 1978). Counseling appears much more effective, however, when the focus is not behavior change but rather changes in decision making, self-acceptance, perceptions of self-efficacy, and other subjectively measured variables (Reynolds, Gutkin, Elliott, & Witt, 1984). Counseling is seen as having a great deal of face validity by educators and administrators, especially since, historically, counseling has been a component of total services offered within public education.

In the study noted earlier by Dustin et al. (1984), school personnel reported they would like even more counseling made available to students, school staff, and parents. Support for counseling extends beyond traditional boundaries for such service in schools to include individual as well as group interventions with students and adults. With such support, professionals engaged in counseling activities must be willing to take a proactive stance to encourage school districts to attach higher priority to counseling services. The need for counseling is great. Consideration of key issues in this text will identify counseling strategies to meet student needs.

OVERVIEW OF THIS BOOK

We will be providing an overview of major approaches to counseling within school settings. Individual as well as group approaches will be examined in terms of goals of counseling, steps to achieve success, and practical implementation issues. Built into the discussion of each option will be how practitioners, whatever their job title, will be able to consider and implement effective counseling interventions.

In addition to focusing on particular approaches, we will consider how the effectiveness of counseling can be evaluated as well as monitored for implementation. Ethical and legal issues will be raised concerning counseling interventions. Finally, we will consider how school practitioners can optimize the effectiveness of counseling within a broader array of services. A number of resources will be identified related to counseling theories, models, and strategies (see Box 1.6).

The reader is encouraged to apply what he/she knows about school systems in making sense of the information presented. Wide variation exists in how practices in counseling are implemented across the United States. Rural settings often differ dramatically from urban settings. Regional differences exist in the focus on psychology versus

BOX 1.6. Practical Concepts from the Four Theories

Each of the four systems offers something concrete for an educator to consider in counseling students. The following chapters will describe specific techniques that will utilize the following:

Rogerian

Relationship developed over time between educator and student

Trust in the student/client

Developing a safe climate for counseling

Focus on feelings

Adlerian

Student learning possible goals for own behavior

Pointing out patterns in child's behavior

Encouragement of student

Enabling logical consequences of behavior to become apparent to the student

Student assuming responsibility for own choices

Behavioral

Clarity of goals between counselor and student

Analyzing situation that surrounds target behavior

Awareness of and provision for reinforcement

Use of contracts

Cognitive behavioral

Understanding of student thinking about and attitudes toward target behaviors

Providing alternative strategies; new ways of thinking, new approaches to problem; and new expectations for student

Cognitive restructuring

---

education within counseling and in who is expected to engage in counseling. Although settings and practitioners will differ, theories and techniques described within this book have had wide application in the United States and surrounding countries. Case studies of individual techniques and strategies will be used to enhance understanding of the variables that can influence eventual effectiveness of counseling.

2

Issues Affecting Counseling

In this chapter the reader is presented with an overview of selected issues that affect counseling interventions in an educational setting. The issues have been selected with a view to their timeliness and because of their direct relevance to those staff members engaging, or about to engage, in counseling interventions in addition to their traditional duties. The issues selected for discussion in this chapter include referring students, counseling as a direct or indirect service, consulting as an intervention compared with counseling, characteristics of schools that can be viewed as barriers and as assets to successful counseling, and those skills that contribute to successful counseling.

REFERRAL CONSIDERATIONS

Referring clients is a process engaged in by all counselors and therapists. Ethical codes indicate the importance of the issue of referrals. Professional counselors are bound to provide services, including counseling, within the limits of their own competency. School practitioners engaging in counseling need to be alert for signs that a client needs another counselor or other services.

When to refer clients is an issue that faces every counselor. There are times when a student/client will present a special type of problem or will display symptoms that were not obvious until several sessions have passed. No counselor has been trained to a level of competence in each type of symptomology that exists. Therefore, each counselor must remain aware of the limits of personal competence and be ready to refer some clients for the specialized help they deserve (see Box 2.1).

At times, as clients communicate deeper and more personal levels of their story, many counselors are plagued by self-doubts.

BOX 2.1. When to Refer

1. You realize that you are not competent to deal with the problem of concern.
2. You are uncertain that you have the time or energy to deal with the student's needs.
3. You prefer *not* to counsel students.
4. A student or a parent asks for a recommendation for counseling.
5. You have initiated counseling, but little has changed for the student, and there is little or no progress.

"Am I able to help this student?" "Should I have become involved? I never thought the client would delve into material like this." Such doubts can be alleviated and tested by consulting with a trusted colleague who has agreed to serve in this capacity *before* the specific doubts begin.

Any school practitioner who engages in counseling with a student should consider obtaining supervision from a colleague. This "supervision" may take the form of frequent consultations with the colleague as the counselor seeks support and ideas about the progress of the couseling.

In addition to the practitioner exceeding limits of competence, a professional may refer a client when the student is not benefiting from the counseling (American Association for Counseling and Development, 1988). Thus, the choice of referring clients is always a possibility for any counselor and can involve formal or informal referral procedures.

Formal Referral Procedures

Professional counseling settings have written guidelines that serve to inform the public how clients come to be served by the organization. Many schools likewise will have some written procedures to be followed when a counselor is referring clients elsewhere for counseling. The reader needs to become informed about the referral procedures, if any, in the specific school being served.

Selecting the referral placement for a particular client is a difficult choice for any counselor. With experience and effort, a counselor comes to develop a list of successful resources for counseling. Some clients require specialized help with such problems as eating disorders, substance abuse, or psychological assessment. Other clients may need group counseling or family counseling. When an individual is making a referral, especially for the first time, considerable affect may be experienced. The counselor may have mixed feelings about the need for a referral. Doubts are common—in spite of the unanimity of ethical guidelines—that "perhaps I *should* be able to help." In addition, there may be feelings of antipathy for the client if the counseling has been frustrating. It is more likely that feelings of concern on the part of the counselor will serve to complicate the referral process. The client's feeling also can be considered. If a warm, trusting relationship exists with a counselor, a client may be reluctant to consider a new service provider.

The helper making the referral, even one following prescribed guidelines when they exist, should plan to stay with the client and to check back in order to determine that satisfactory service is being provided. The counselor can refer the client to a specific individual in an agency and follow up to ensure that contact has occurred (see Box 2.2).

Counselors providing services in schools are also faced with the common occurrence that clients are often minors and may be regarded as not capable of making some decisions on their own. Nevertheless, the guidelines for referral still apply, even though an adult will sometimes be needed to successfully complete certain referrals. People regarded as minors must be granted the right to competent counseling and to counseling that is satisfactorily accomplishing something. The client must not have his/her privacy invaded when the counselor is working with a parent or guardian to achieve a successful referral.

For example, Ms. Smith agreed to meet with Audrey Taylor, a parent of one of her fifth graders. However, Mrs. Taylor needed more time-consuming attention than Ms. Smith had to give. Therefore, Ms. Smith, after consulting with her principal, called the school district's social worker and informed her that she was going to refer a parent. Then at their next scheduled meeting, Ms. Smith expressed her concern for Mrs. Taylor and informed her that the school dis-

---

BOX 2.2. How to Refer

---

1. Consult with a colleague regarding the best course of action.
2. When referring "in house," contact the counselor to discuss your recommendations.
3. When referring to a community agency, provide choices for the student and parents. Identify two or three professionals whom you know to be skilled in dealing with the problem of concern.
4. Follow up your recommendation to confirm that contact has been made.

Note: Verify school policies concerning referrals before proceeding.

trict's social worker would be better suited to work with her. Ms. Smith gave Mrs. Taylor the number to call, offered to call the social worker right then to schedule an appointment, and told Mrs. Taylor that she would be glad to meet with her about her daughter, Lottie Taylor, even if Mrs. Taylor herself met with the social worker.

School psychologists and school social workers in many school districts work under specific restrictions in dealing with minors. For example, written parental permission may be required before the professional can even meet with the student to discuss problems. When referral to an outside agency is considered, the parent would similarly be asked to permit the recommended service. Counselors and teachers often can make suggestions about recommended services directly to the student. A wise policy for any school practitioner is to check before making referrals for any school district policies concerning parental permission.

Informal Referral Procedures

Crucially important for a successful referral are the informal techniques for making a client feel comfortable and assured that a referral is in the client's best interest. For example, each staff member in an educational setting can begin to determine which referrals—that is, which therapists, clinics, and counseling centers—seem to be the most highly regarded by counselors and by former clients. This informal assessment is a godsend when a harried professional seeks to help someone who seems in desperate need of effective counseling. Additionally, within the neighboring community of each school, there will be frequent open houses or public events that would allow the educator to get inside an agency and begin to assess the climate, warmth, type of clientele, and other factors relevant for a successful referral.

Finally, a trusted colleague can be an excellent source of information about possibilities for a referral. It is important to remember that if the educator provides a choice for the client or the client's parents, then the choice is theirs. The educator does not often make the final decision for someone else. But the counselor who is involved is in a crucial position to support the client in this most important decision of where to seek further help. Many counselors provide the client or family with service choices, allowing free and informed consent during all stages of a referral.

Informal referrals differ from formal ones in that there might not be specified steps to follow. For example, the professional educator might communicate concern to the parent. "I am very concerned about what you have been telling me. I believe your problem calls for some specialized help. I know you want to do the right thing for Lottie, your fifth grader, and I believe you should find a counselor who can spend the time with you to help you resolve this situation. I just don't have the time. What are your reactions to my suggestion?"

After considering the parent's reaction, the educator would want to provide at least two resources for the parent to consider. The resources that are recommended would be known to the educator either by reputation or through past contact.

COUNSELING AS A DIRECT OR INDIRECT SERVICE

Many of the educational functions within a school can be viewed as direct services. Examples include teaching, supervising, delivering food to students and staff, and several other necessary functions. Counseling can be viewed as another of these direct services. Direct services occur between the provider and the recipient. Direct services almost always include some goals or outcomes to be achieved between the two parties, the student learning in the case of teaching or advice and feedback provided to the supervisee in the case of supervision.

Counseling is usually viewed as a direct service. The helper interacts face to face with the client. Although the client's goals for counseling will almost always be directed at situations outside the counseling office (for example, problems with friends or in a class), nevertheless, counseling usually includes some immediate goals such as helping the student feel better or to resolve an uncertainty.

Indirect services also occur in educational settings (see Box 2.3). Functions that involve a third party, an intermediary, or that are directed at long-range goals are often described as indirect. Preventive activities therefore will often be indirect. For example, staff members who engage in orientation activities are engaging in services that have an impact in the middle- or long-range future. Helping new students anticipate problems *before* they enroll is another example of

BOX 2.3. Direct versus Indirect Services

Direct services	Indirect services
Hands-on contact with student (one-to-one arrangement)	Work with staff members who then work with student
Time-intensive	Time-efficient
Help prepare student for specific needs	Help prepare staff to work with many students
Counseling services (individual or group), teaching	Consulting and other interventions, workshops

preventive service. Showing students their lockers and allowing them to walk around the building when school begins can help alleviate problems later.

When a staff member listens to a student, many educators would label the activity a part of a direct service, teaching. When the staff member listens to the student outside of class time and alone in a classroom, some would still include this as a part of teaching, although a very personal, or even unusual, part. When the student, alone with a caring, concerned teacher, shifts the topic away from school work to the loneliness of attending the particular school, an exact label cannot be attached to the teacher's role. In many such instances, the educator can use selected aspects of counseling in order to maximize the teacher's use of time and help accomplish goals with the student.

Teachers and other staff members who engage in the activity of counseling are providing indirect services when they are serving to improve the learning capability of the student and improve the climate of the entire school. The availability of staff willing to listen and to become involved with students in need adds a positive element to school services. Most such counseling activities by educational staff members will be situational in nature and short term. School practitioners without the job title of "counselor" will seldom stop to analyze whether their actions are a direct or indirect service. They will instead focus on their primary objective of helping the student in need.

COUNSELING VERSUS CONSULTING

Two services that can be viewed as direct or indirect, depending on the circumstances, are consulting and counseling. Although this text is designed to describe in some detail counseling services, consulting is a practical service that may prove to be a helpful alternative for some educators.

Consulting has been described as a three-party helping process (Dustin & Blocher, 1984). The help seeker is named the *consultee*. When the help seeker is having difficulty with a third party, the *client*, then the consulting process can help the consultee improve problem-solving skills.

Although many models and consulting processes have been presented elsewhere (Brown, Pryzwansky, & Schulte, 1987; Gallessich, 1982), consultation can be described as a problem-solving process in which the helper, the *consultant*, helps the consultee to proceed systematically through a series of problem-solving stages. Consultees may be students who are having troubles with other students or with teachers, or parents concerned about their own children, or other teachers. The consultant very carefully focuses on the fact that the person seeking help has the problem and that the consultant does not need to assume the problem as his/her own. Stages of consulting will be considered as follows:

Defining the Problem

The consultant begins the helping process by assisting the help seeker to define the difficulty that caused the problem. Often, just the clarification of a difficulty is viewed as extremely helpful by the consultee. Usually, the help seeker is having difficulty with students or with another staff member. At this stage, the helper can focus the conversation to get the consultee to specify just what it is about the situation that is the most troubling. Helping the consultee specify the difficulty is the most important aspect of this first stage.

Considering Alternative Solutions

After the problem is specified, the consultant assists the consultee to list some alternatives that could alleviate the problem. Rather than proposing one idea or solution, the consultant can help the consultee actually consider many options. This is done most directly by helping the consultee list more than one possibility of how to deal with the problem.

Selecting and Implementing a Solution

After the consultee has selected a strategy for solving the difficulty, the work of the consultant includes checking back and giving support to the consultee as the plan is carried out. In those cases in which the selected solution takes care of the difficulty, the process can proceed to the evaluation step.

However, as might be expected, there will be instances when the consultee will not experience immediate success. Then, as with any problem-solving process, the consultant encourages the consultee to return to the problem definition stage. Has the entire problem been described? Is the exact problem the one focused on during the earlier consulting? Then a return to considering alternative solutions is needed. At times additional solutions will be discovered. Perhaps the consultee needs to do some reading or receive training or acquire experience in implementing a solution. At any rate, the consultation leads to the selection of another, more refined solution, and once again the consultant becomes a source of support to the consultee.

Evaluation

It is highly recommended that each educator who engages in the consultant role check back with the consultee in order to engage in a mutual evaluation of the process, including such topics as the helpfulness of the consultant, the ultimate outcome of the activity, and the behavior of the client. Although this is easy enough to overlook in the bustle of real educational service delivery, educators can gain expertise and add to their effectiveness if they will bother to evaluate their efforts as a consultant.

Termination

It is important to signal the end of the consultation process. As envisioned here, consultation is a service provided at school between two parties who are dealing with a school-related problem. Therefore, it seems important that consultation be considered by the educator who is approached for help while on the job. Since the regular duties of the two parties will no doubt require interaction about other concerns and day-to-day interactions, it will be less confusing for both parties to agree that a specific consultation is ended.

The consultation process possesses some advantages over counseling. The necessary skills and the clear step-by-step nature of the service make it attractive for many educators. In addition, consultation has the advantage of designating that the one with the problem is the consultee. At times the counseling process serves to involve the helper to such an extent that this person assumes much of the responsibility for the symptoms of the help seeker. This is easy for a caring educator to do. Consultation is less likely than counseling to result in the school practitioner assuming ownership of the help seeker's problem.

Finally, consultation has the advantage of flexibility. For example, the help seeker could be a student. The educator may be able to help the student specify just which third party, often a parent or a teacher, is giving the student difficulty and then proceed through the other stages of consultation.

An example can differentiate a teacher's consulting from counseling (Box 2.4). Recall that in an earlier example, Ms. Smith was starting to counsel Audrey Taylor.

After Ms. Smith referred Mrs. Taylor to the district social worker for counseling, Mrs. Taylor got a divorce. Now, later in the same school year, Ms. Smith is listening to Mrs. Taylor describe the fifth grade daughter's difficulties adjusting to the divorce. Note that the

BOX 2.4. Counseling versus Consulting

Counseling	Consulting
Relationship with student—direct contact with client)	Relationship with staff—no direct client contact
Individual or group focus	Usually individual focus
Emphasis on student's coping	Emphasis on staff's coping
Affective and cognitive	Cognitive
Long or short term	Short term
Student commits to action	Staff commits to action

problem involves a third party, Lottie. As Ms. Smith helps define the problem, Lottie's refusal to do homework, she and Mrs. Taylor consider some alternatives. Mrs. Taylor decides on a plan that will involve Ms. Smith praising Lottie and sending notes home when the homework is done. The role of Ms. Smith is to check back with Mrs. Taylor, the consultee, and listen to Mrs. Taylor's satisfaction with the plan. The goal of Ms. Smith is to provide a short-term service (consulting) that will enhance the parent's problem-solving skills (see Box 2.5), *not* to engage in a long-term counseling arrangement that might influence Mrs. Taylor's affective status.

School psychologists and school social workers frequently consult with other school practitioners as well as parents and students. In schools not served by a full-time psychologist or social worker, consulting may be the strategy of choice in providing help. A major advantage of consultation is that it allows the professional the opportunity to work on a problem *without* offering direct services to the client. With increased problem-solving skills, the consultee initiates the change process, and the professional remains available as a resource for ideas and as an objective evaluator.

BARRIERS AND ASSETS TO COUNSELING

As mentioned in the introduction, schools vary, and each educational setting is unique. Therefore, the reader will need to apply the follow-

BOX 2.5. Stages of Consulting

1. Information gathering: "What is the presenting problem?"
2. Diagnosis: "What is causing the problem?"
3. Planning and implementation: "What can we do?"
4. Evaluation: "What happened?"

ing characteristics that are described as impinging on successful counseling to the individual school being served. Certain characteristics of schools may be viewed as barriers, although not insurmountable, to appropriate delivery of counseling to needy students. A few such characteristics are mentioned below to stimulate the readers' awareness and thinking about whether similar factors exist for them.

Turf issues are frequently a basis for heated, and sometimes long-lasting, discussions or even conflicts within an educational institution. Providers of certain services may resent apparent intrusion into "their" area.

Such disturbances often continue within the levels of authority until an administrative decision is made that either allows or forbids the service that has been seen as intruding into the area of another service provider. For example, a school with several counselors, a school psychologist, and a school social worker may experience conflict over who should be delivering each service. Each professional may feel qualified to counsel students but resent the intrusion of other professionals into the area regarded as his/her specialty. Districts with detailed policies on service providers can eliminate some of the conflict over turf, but often negotiation is necessary to deal with differences in the perceptions of who should be doing what.

In addition, it is possible that a staff member who is not titled a counselor, psychologist, or social worker but who engages in actively listening to students may be viewed as infringing on the turf of professional support staff. However, the need exists for some adult figure in many educational settings to be available to listen to a particular student at a specific time of need when the student chooses to disclose a problem. Administrators and teachers will often choose to work, using counseling techniques, with students who seem in special need of attention.

In many educational settings, the expectations that students have of school staff will be quite specific, even rigid. Students, and perhaps other staff and family members, may have developed quite strong ideas about which employees will be available to listen to the troubled student. Even expectations of staff members become quite strong about what is expected and even what is tolerated in the schools. We do not envision any staff members setting up counseling services as an alternative to or in competition with existing services. Rather, it is our experience that many staff members are already perceived as understanding and trustworthy people with whom students want to talk about personal problems. Within any school, however, individual staff members may react to the notion of counseling students by saying, "that is not my job," or perhaps, "someone else is supposed to listen to students."

Even more of a barrier is the common lament of educators—time. With the demands of modern society being imposed on schools seemingly without end, many staff members have no doubt already wondered when they "are supposed to find time" to listen to students (see Box 2.6).

Another barrier to effective counseling is the isolation of staff members, so common in many schools. Physical distance, scattered schedules, and constant activity and movement may present a very real barrier to a chance for some staff to offer thoughtful, private, quiet attention to a needy student.

None of the barriers described here will automatically go away, but the seeming fact that the most competent staff members in educational settings are given the most to do is very real. Schools will differ in how difficult barriers to counseling students are to be overcome.

Fortunately, there are several factors that function as assets to motivate staff members to provide counseling in the schools. The students themselves seek out and reinforce the staff member who decides to provide a listening relationship. The obvious needs of so many students help many busy staff members decide to become involved. In addition, the openness and trusting nature of many students often result in a caring staff member being drawn into a counseling-like relationship before any decision is overtly made to act as a counselor.

In addition, many staff members are located physically close to students, include daily or frequent contact, and call for ongoing communication, which allows close, open relationships to develop. Some professional providers of counseling with little daily contact with students have to spend time and attempt to develop trust and familiarity with concerns before being comfortable with students. The daily concerns can include scheduling problems such as wanting to drop a class. Guidance surveys of adolescent students historically have shown that many students turn to friends, parents, teach-

BOX 2.6. Personal Barriers and Assets to Counseling

Barriers	Assets
Personal time and energy	Challenge of helping others
Colleagues' perception of role	Student's perceptions of you
Administrative support	Collegial support
Training	Student and parent expectations
Student and parent expectations	Satisfaction of helping others

ers, and coaches for advice and help with personal concerns. Frequent contact allows relationships to begin before students ask for help.

An asset that can influence a school practitioner to engage in counseling lies in the availability of concerned caring colleagues. There is always a professional staff member within the acquaintance of the educator who cares enough to provide consultation and supervision to the staff member who begins to listen to a student in need. Availability of support means that the educator who is acquainted with the barriers described above can still become involved since advice and support are available.

Finally, another important asset to effective counseling can be found in the skills possessed by the educational staff. In order to be successful as a teacher or other staff member, school practitioners must already possess effective communication skills. With support and feedback from colleagues, an educator's abilities can result in a counseling intervention that is likely to be helpful.

An example concerns John, a student in a vocational high school, and his welding instructor, Mr. Earl. John started talking to Mr. Earl about the chances of obtaining a job using his welding skills. However, their discussion quickly turned to John's unhappiness with his girlfriend.

Mr. Earl knew that the counselors in the school would not worry about their "turf" being violated if he talked with John about his problems. In fact, Mr. Earl consulted with one of the counselors as he met with John over the course of a few weeks. In addition, although he didn't consider himself an expert, Mr. Earl didn't mind John beginning to talk about his girl. In fact, Mr. Earl thought that John's emotional state helped explain the recent change in John's work. Finally, although conditions were very noisy, Mr. Earl held his discussion with John in the shop area, where both were working. During their discussion, Mr. Earl tried to listen carefully and to not interrupt John. When talk centered on John's feelings about being rejected, Mr. Earl listened carefully and used some of the skills discussed in the next section.

SKILLS CONTRIBUTING TO SUCCESSFUL COUNSELING

Although much of the knowledge and many of the life skills possessed by each staff member can be used to help students seeking a helpful listener, four sets of skills contribute to successful counseling within any educational institution. Additional listening skills are described in later chapters on individual and group counseling.

Friendliness

The demeanor of the educator with an above average chance to provide successful counseling to needy students will no doubt include friendliness. Whether stemming from an inborn sense of optimism or reflecting an inner sense of self-worth, the friendly, optimistic educator will more likely be sought out by students than will the resident grump. We can become aware of our demeanor as we hurry in the halls, arrive at crowded doorways in the mornings, and pass through students on our way to the car after school. How likely is it that we project a warmth or an approachability that indicates that we are someone who could be helpful to students?

Trustworthiness

The grapevine among students will have a lot to say about whether the educator is viewed as someone who can be trusted. Whenever a person turns to another to share a problem, whether a trusted friend or a professional, there is an expectation that this person will not use what is disclosed against the person in need. Students are especially susceptible to breach of confidentiality since so many schools have norms that anything can be discussed in the lounge or that anything a student discloses in class is fair game for gossip. Successful counseling requires that the client can trust that any information will only be used for the client's benefit. Practitioner skills that help build trust include genuineness and self-disclosure (Box 2.7). The importance of these skills is demonstrated in later chapters.

Humor

The educator who possesses a sense of humor and who is able to see the lighter side of even dark moments is more likely than other colleagues to persevere and to succeed in helping needy students. Although humor is two-edged and can be abused, nevertheless, the ability to laugh at oneself and to maintain perspective in even critical moments is likely to help counseling succeed.

BOX 2.7. Practicing the Skills of Genuineness and Self-Disclosure

This exercise suggests ways of practicing genuineness and self-disclosure. Opportunity for feedback is provided. Four persons are required for the complete set of activities, which can be used with adults or students.

GOALS

1. To increase understanding of genuineness and self-disclosure.
2. To stimulate practice of the skills.
3. To provide feedback on use of the two skills.

DIRECTIONS

Practice Self-Disclosure

a. Select a partner. Take turns practicing self-disclosures. For example, share an interest, hobby, or experience. Ask whether your remarks are clear.

b. Add a third person. With one of you acting as observer, make additional self-disclosures and have the third person paraphrase what is heard. Check with the observer: Was the self-disclosure clear? How accurate was the paraphrase? Change roles and repeat the exercise.

Practice Genuineness

In groups of three, assign roles (speaker, listener, observer). Speaker tells listener a story that contains two or more statements of feeling in a given situation (for example, "I was so mad when he said that"). The listener then restates the feelings being expressed (reflecting feelings). The observer then assesses the clarity of the feeling statements (were they concise?) and the accuracy of the restatement. Participants exchange roles and continue.

Practice of Both Skills

a. Form two partnerships. Using the *Partner Observation Form,* tally all genuine and self-disclosing statements made by your partner. Exchange roles and continue.

b. Partners can be exchanged to continue practice.

Practice on Videotape

The skills of self-disclosure and genuiness are especially good to practice on videotape, allowing you to observe your nonverbal behaviors. You can work alone or with a partner to assess the use of skills related to self-disclosure and genuineness.

(continued)

BOX 2.7. (*Continued*)

PARTNER OBSERVATION FORM

Name: _____

Partner's name: _____

Directions: Record the genuine feelings expressed by your partner. Describe nonverbal behaviors evident while partner is speaking. Below, write self-disclosure statements, whether length of statement appears too long or about right, and your reactions to the statement.

Genuineness   Nonverbal behavior _____

1.
2.
3.
4.
5.

Self-disclosure statement   Length   Your reaction

1.
2.
3.
4.
5.

Other observations of partner _____

Being System-Wise

This descriptor is not a single skill but a series of skills about the educational setting in which the counseling occurs and will certainly help counseling succeed. Knowledge about the entire educational system, the specific school, but also about all the support agencies and other schools is an important asset that few students have on their own. The staff member who is familiar with the power structure, and especially the informal power structure within the building and throughout the educational system, is in a unique position to help students with certain problems.

Familiarity with the communication system is an asset that may help counseling result in successful outcomes for a client. Just who talks to whom? With whom is the registrar or the assistant principal most likely to discuss the new schedule?

The counselor may elect to refer students to other students, to clubs, or to sponsors of certain activities. Knowledge about all facets of the system is included in the descriptor, *system-wise*. In addition to providing a listening ear, successful counselors also need to provide accurate information at times in order to achieve success.

In short, there are many issues that contribute to the effectiveness of counseling offered by professional school practitioners. Important issues about when to become involved and when to refer students to others were described in this chapter. Throughout the chapter the reader was directed to consider the many needs of students and the likelihood that some students will prefer to talk to an instructor or to someone they know. Interested staff can help such students and can collaborate to offer services based on their strengths. Many staff are interested in students and, while recognizing their own limitations of knowledge and of time, have an important role to play in using counseling techniques to serve students.

3

Individual Counseling

Counseling the individual student can influence important aspects of how a school-age child thinks and feels. The school practitioner, whether the school psychologist, counselor, social worker, teacher, or administrator, will face children in need of attention and individualized care. Professionals, with sufficient preparation and experience, can guide students toward more productive actions at school and home and can assist students to solve problems that occur outside of the direct supervision of adults.

How does the school practitioner decide which student needs individual attention or when counseling is the strategy of choice? This chapter addresses both of these questions. The reader will see that many children are in need of individual attention and that counseling will be recommended for several types of problems that children report. We will emphasize that counseling a child in a one-on-one arrangement requires specific skills, preparation for meetings, and regular evaluation.

What skills are needed for the practitioner interested in working with individual students? Professional codes of ethics typically specify that a practitioner must have responsibility for and competence in all aspects of services delivered. Minimum preparation to call oneself a *counselor* will entail, as might be expected, formal training in counseling theory and practices. Many professionals in schools, on the other hand, can argue with justification that they deliver counseling services without a degree in counseling. Psychologists, social workers, and other educators may provide individual care to students that an outsider might label counseling.

In this chapter, we assume that the reader delivers or is interested in delivering services that could be considered counseling and that sufficient preparation to provide such services has included some formal exposure to the topic, some experience in counseling students on an individual basis, and interest in acquiring more knowledge and expertise in services to children. To call oneself a counselor will be distinguished from performing services defined as counseling.

PROBLEMS ADDRESSED BY COUNSELING

A number of student behaviors can surface in the school setting and lead to a referral for individual counseling. As noted in previous chapters, the need for individual attention for children has been reported by both school practitioners and students. Parents also request individual attention regarding their concerns for their children and their ability to function as parents. Counseling can be directed to assist students or parents to deal more effectively with personal issues that either interfere with functioning or limit ability to experience success (Box 3.1).

A student's age relates to the types of issues or problems that surface during counseling. Adolescents are more likely than younger children to seek support for peer-related difficulties, academic prob-

---

BOX 3.1. Issues in Counseling Children

Factors that influence focus on individual counseling
    Type of problem (for example, school-related, home-related)
    Nature of problem (for example, relations with peers)
    Urgency of need (for example, crisis?)
    Age of student (elementary, secondary)
    Willingness of student (voluntary, requested by adult)
    Inner-directed or outer-directed problem (passive, aggressive)

Girls seek counseling for the following
    Passive behaviors
    Peer relations (girlfriends, boyfriends)

Boys seek counseling for the following
    Problems with teachers (academics)
    Problems with aggression (discipline)

Practitioners initiate offer to counsel child when
    Approached by student
    Are aware of problems and experience concern
    Implement a proactive or preventive program
    Colleagues suggest need to talk
    Parents suggest talk with child

---

lems (especially related to the student's postsecondary plans), and assistance in dealing with parents or community agents (the latter if the child is involved with nonschool programs such as juvenile justice agency activities or is looking for help in finding work). Preadolescents in elementary schools or junior highs may need help in understanding adult expectations for behavior or guidance on how to behave around classmates. Any child involved in what an adult might label a crisis (usually relating to family life) can benefit from support from a caring professional.

Boys and girls appear with differing frequencies for counseling services. Girls are much more likely than boys to be considered for counseling for inner-directed or passive behaviors such as shyness and self-consciousness. Stone (1981) reviews the types of problems considered by teachers to be problems. Most boys escape the attention of a teacher for negative behaviors, but several activities have a high likelihood of being labeled a problem by teachers. High-frequency items include the following: restlessness, distractability, disruptiveness, inattentiveness, disobedience, fighting, and other externally directed behaviors. Whether such actions merit a counseling intervention will depend on the teacher's, student's, and support professional's attempts to modify behaviors via direct intervention based in the classroom. Generally, a problem behavior will occur over a period of time and be resistant to classroom interventions before counseling is elected as the strategy of choice.

School practitioners with daily student contact will observe a variety of patterns of classroom behaviors. Most students will present a consistent "face" to the world. When behaviors vary from the expected, adults become alerted to possible difficulties in the child's life. The school practitioner has the immediate option of talking with the student about present events or of referring the child to someone who has sufficient rapport to draw out the student's feelings and perceptions. Some students will not wait for adult attention but will approach a trusted teacher or staff member to discuss concerns. By whatever means the student and school practitioner link up, the decision remains about what to do about the student's problems— whether to help through counseling, refer the child to another professional, or let the student deal with the issues alone.

The parent may be involved in affirming the need for counseling. As noted in Chapter 2, school psychologists and other professionals may be required to secure parental permission before providing a service. Other school practitioners, at times, may seek out information from the parent to better understand a student's account of problems. In such instances, confidentiality between the student and practitioner will be a concern, as we will address later. Issues being discussed by a 6-year-old and a 16-year-old will elicit, in general, different approaches from the staff member and differing concerns about the need for parental involvement. The staff member providing individual counseling may contact the parent for a conference to review both the reasons for counseling and the agenda that counseling can cover with the child. Some parents will insist on having the opportunity to review the school's case for services before indicating willingness to have their child participate in counseling. The child's input is always relevant to the decision on whether to offer individual counseling.

Consider the junior high student who has been referred by a classroom teacher to the assistant principal. Hector has been doing well in the class (social studies) for the past semester but lately seems distracted. The quality of his work has deteriorated, and his grades have confirmed that he is having difficulty. The teacher was convinced that possibly events at home (primarily the marital problems of the parents) were to blame but did not want to discuss home life with Hector. The assistant principal, a former counselor, had success talking to students and motivating them in their studies. Hector, on the other hand, proved to have no interest in being counseled by the administrator and reacted angrily when the subject of his family was raised. He was quite vehement in wanting to be left alone. Two weeks later, Hector approached his teacher and asked to talk about what he could do about his grades. He stated that he wanted to do well because he liked the class but didn't want to be sent to the assistant principal who was "nosy." The teacher consulted with the assistant principal to see what she could do for Hector. The administrator reviewed what he had attempted and checked to see if the teacher was interested in working with Hector on his current problems. When the teacher affirmed her interest, the assistant principal provided direction and ongoing feedback to the teacher as she counseled the student about his concerns. With guidance from the teacher, Hector seemed better able to satisfy in-class expectations.

Students appreciate being involved in decisions that affect them, such as being asked about whether they would be willing to become involved in counseling. Participation in the decision to counsel can increase the student's commitment to work during and outside of sessions. Students often work harder when they see what their investment of time and energy will produce. Respect for the student translates, at times, into extended discussions in which the school practitioner and the student define the scope and content of counseling sessions. A formal (contract) or informal agreement may be the result, so that both participants have an idea of the extent and details of services and how information generated will be disseminated. The goals of counseling will be defined after the participants agree that continuing individual attention will be the intervention of choice.

GOALS OF COUNSELING

Once an agreement is reached that counseling will assist the student, the goals of counseling can be clarified by participants. The individual counseling approach is attractive to school practitioners for several reasons. Only one student may appear to be in need of service, or the practitioner has only the time and energy for the individual child. When extensive resources are available within the school, individual counseling may be selected by staff based on a commitment to individual attention and a determination that the student will be receptive to services. Some students do not want to participate in groups. Displays of shyness or excessive aggressiveness can convince the staff to work individually with the student to teach specific communication and social skills. On the other hand, staff can elect to enroll shy and aggressive students in groups with the express purpose of shaping new behaviors. Chapters 5 and 6 review group counseling alternatives for students.

As noted in Chapter 1, an important goal of counseling is to teach specific skills to students. Yet this goal cannot be achieved until the staff member responsible for counseling is able to motivate the student to express concerns or perceptions related to current behaviors. Early stages of individual counseling sessions can be devoted to developing an atmosphere of trust and caring, especially when the school practitioner and the student do not know each other well. Staff members who are not assigned full time to a building, such as a school psychologist or social worker, will need time to build rapport with the student. In one school, a school psychologist had an informal policy of visiting each classroom at least once a month, speaking to any class on invitation, and attending as many student events as possible so that every student had a chance to observe her. When students came for counseling, the psychologist was not considered a stranger. Time was still needed to shape trust to the level necessary for counseling, but the major hurdle of familiarity had been overcome. Setting goals became an opportunity for the psychologist to display awareness of what was occurring in the school and individual classrooms.

Several writers have provided suggestions for counseling goals during the work of individual counseling (Box 3.2). George and Cristiani

(1986), for example, list five major priorities of the counseling process. The five include facilitating behavior change, enhancing coping skills, promoting decision making, improving relationships, and facilitating client potential. The expression of these goals may involve some overlap, as the counselor and child can pursue the development of new behaviors that affect the child's success within several areas. How the practitioner works to achieve these goals will vary along several dimensions, including the help giver's theoretical orientation, available time, nature of the presenting problem, and abilities of the client.

Neely (1982) proposes an additional goal for special education students. She considers normalization, the process by which the handicapped student acquires skills that allow for integration into the regular classroom, an important emphasis of counseling. Motivation of special needs students so that they can benefit from counseling is an important concern for practitioners. The reader who works with handicapped students is encouraged to seek out Neely's text for an excellent overview of special counseling practices.

The time that the student and practitioner spend discussing and setting goals allows both parties to see how the other thinks and acts. The two can reflect on whether counseling is the best direction to take for now, given the student's concerns, and can clarify the student's motivation to deal with presenting problems. The practitioner can further assess whether a more highly skilled counselor would be better able to handle the student and his/her concerns.

BOX 3.2. Goals of Individual Counseling

Facilitating behavior change
Enhancing coping skills
Promoting decision making
Improving relationships
Facilitating client potential
    —George and Cristiani (1986)

Normalization for handicapped students—relations with nonhandicapped peers and the realities of the regular classroom
    —Neely (1982)

Motivate students to express concerns related to behaviors
Help students accept responsibility for behavior
Train students in specific skills (for example, study skills, homework)
    —Ehly and Dustin

Facilitating Behavior Change

The child's behavior often will be the primary force motivating consideration of counseling services. As noted above, acting-out behaviors comprise the majority of referrals from teachers for formal services. On the other hand, shy and withdrawn behaviors can lead to a referral, especially in those cases when these behaviors represent a shift from previous patterns. Targeting specific behaviors for change can be relatively straightforward. If, for example, Mr. Sparks, a teacher, is concerned about Ron's ongoing difficulties in relating to peers, counseling can be considered to develop the student's social skills.

When to refer or consider for counseling will vary with the school setting and the practitioner. In many schools, experienced counselors are readily available and are trusted by students. Often, teachers will consider referral when the student is perceived to be experiencing some difficulty that staff members are prepared, as part of their assignment, to address. Thus, problems and concerns of the student, whether related to school or not, can be considered as a basis for referral. Some schools will even advertise availability of counseling services for students.

In some instances, the staff member will consider his/her own willingness to work individually with the student. Some students will seek out a particular teacher and express openness for help *only* from that person. Whatever staff member sees the child in need of attention, the key elements of a decision to counsel will be relevant expertise, time and energy, and a commitment from the student to talk.

Setting goals and planning activities for counseling sessions can vary with the counseling model followed by practitioners. Behavioral models refine goal statements so that an independent observer can verify characteristics of problem behaviors and confirm progress toward behavior change goals set by the student and the school practitioner. Other models, such as the Rogerian and Adlerian approaches, can result in goals that more openly consider changes in feelings, attitudes, and thoughts. As might be expected, how the goal is stated will relate directly to how change is evaluated. Changes in observable behaviors can be assessed by watching the child, whereas changes in feelings, attitudes, and thoughts will involve asking the child for information.

Enhancing Coping Skills

Coping skills reflect two broad dimensions of events, which can be labeled normative and nonnormative. Normative events consist of the daily circumstances that affect all human beings, such as relating to others, conducting all tasks necessary for success in society, and all other everyday occurrences. Attending school, experiencing the pressures of the classroom, and relating to parents would qualify as normative events.

Nonnormative events are those special circumstances that can lead to extra demands on a child's resources in coping. Natural disasters, family tragedies, unexpected happenings (for example, winning a million dollars in the state lottery) can introduce strains to the child and the family. Although we would all like to win the state lottery, such occurrences are unlikely. Much more common are those situations that introduce conflict and stress into the child's world.

Whether demands on the child's coping skills are normative or nonnormative, the practitioner can develop counseling goals that reflect the child's needs and resources. Working to help a child become a better problem solver or better test taker can enhance coping skills. Working with the child under extreme stress related to a nonnormative event can be labeled "crisis intervention" and involve many of the skills discussed in this text. Whatever the circumstances that lead to working with the student, the school practitioner will opt for a counseling intervention when goals set for change require intensive individual work with the student to produce changes in affect and behavior.

Promoting Decision Making

When children have difficulty in identifying options for behavior and considering the consequences of their choices, the practitioner may focus on promoting decision making during individual sessions with the client. Adolescents often report having difficulty in understanding and mastering the decisions facing them as they move closer to adult status. Havighurst (1951) noted several developmental tasks that could, indeed, complicate the decision-making process for adolescents. Facing the adolescent are the following tasks: "(1) accepting one's physique and sexual role; (2) establishing new peer relationships with both sexes; (3) achieving emotional independence from parents; (4) achieving assurance of economic independence; (5) selecting and preparing for an occupation; (6) developing intellectual skills and concepts necessary for civic competence; (7) acquiring socially responsible behavior patterns; (8) preparing for marriage and family life; (9) building conscious values that are harmonious with one's environment" (Prout & Brown, 1983, p. 13).

Inherent to these areas are the decisions necessary to identify and

act on choices of behavior. The practitioner with a preventive orientation can consider such goals with younger children, working to prepare them for the choice points of adolescence and young adulthood.

Improving Relationships

The goals of counseling often focus on improving relationships, as
might be expected given such previous goals as facilitating behavior
change and enhancing coping skills. Whether children have problems
relating to peers, adults, or both, the goals of counseling can center on
helping the child to become more successful in relating to others. One
facet of working toward this goal can be to focus on the student's
motivation or desire to behave in such a way that more success is
experienced in relationships with peers and adults.

Teachers may have educational goals for the child that relate to
interpersonal skills. The child who prefers to work alone and seems
lost in group activities may need some training in communicating with
peers. Similarly, the child who has essential interpersonal skills and
needs practice in using them in new situations can benefit from
counseling. Working within a group setting can assist many children,
although others will first need to work on an individual basis to
acquire or practice specific skills successfully before being integrated
into a setting with peers.

Facilitating Client Potential

The final area of counseling goals sounds very broad but can be
considered under two dimensions proposed by Blocher (1966).
Counseling can assist the child to realize personal limitations as well as
the realities of the home and school environment. Children can become frustrated when they realize that their actions or preferences
result in consequences from the "real world." The child, for example,
who is capable but does not like to study can be counseled on what is
needed to achieve personal goals (for example, law school) and
guided toward resources that can help him/her manage time and
energy to complete the education and preparation needed to achieve
such goals.

Counseling can be addressed, additionally, to maximize the child's
control over the environment and how he/she identifies and manages
resources. Skills involved in control include many covered in the
other goal areas. The child or adolescent may have difficulty making
sense of the world around him/her. The everyday stresses of childhood can lead to difficulties for even capable children to organize

their lives and make choices that keep them out of trouble and in control of their environment. Extreme examples of difficulties in coping, such as alcoholism and drug abuse, may require special attention much more intensive than a broader counseling program aimed at helping the student to develop perceptions of self-control. Similarly, threats or attempts of suicide should elicit a heightened degree of intervention by the school and family.

Whatever goals are developed, the practitioner and the student can agree on additional issues such as the timing of activities and how information will be handled. (The issue of confidentiality is addressed in other sections of this text.) The goals of counseling will have a direct bearing on how the counselor and client proceed in their contacts.

STEPS IN THE COUNSELING PROCESS

The option of individual counseling can involve a general series of steps or phases that require consideration by the practitioner (Box 3.3). Although the theoretical orientation of the professional can influence the expression of the steps, actions with the client will follow a common pattern. Assuming that permission for counseling has been secured and ground rules for the sessions have been specified (for example, the contract for service, including issues of confidentiality and mechanics of meetings), the practitioner will address the following issues: (1) problem identification (review of the presenting problem and assessment of client needs); (2) problem analysis (consideration of issues relevant to the supporting problem); (3) therapeutic/educational/training applications (activities that involve the client in concerted change); (4) evaluation of change activities; and (5) assisting the client to generalize skills back to the classroom or home.

Identification of the Problem

The child who approaches a practitioner for service can present diverse needs. As many adults are aware, the issues raised by the student for the staff member's attention can vary dramatically from the content of eventual counseling.

Consider Melinda, who, with the support of her teacher, met with Ms. Sykes, her former teacher, to talk about what was on her mind. Melinda, at age 14, had been an average student and popular with peers until the current school year. Events at home, according to the

---
BOX 3.3. Steps in Individual Problem Solving

Problem identification
  Review of the present problem
  Assessment of client needs

Problem analysis
  Consideration of issues and behaviors relevant to problem
  Development of a plan of action (strategy and tactics)

Therapeutic/educational/training intervention
  Implement activities to change client

Evaluation of change program
  Monitor implementation
  Assess outcomes

Assist client to generalize behaviors
  Train client to recognize appropriate use of skills
  Monitor generalization and follow up on applications

---

school's grapevine, were disrupting Melinda's ability to deal with the pressures of school.

Ms. Sykes fully expected to hear Melinda talk about problems at home. Ms. Sykes's first words, "Tell me what's on your mind," were intended to get Melinda to describe events related to current problems in school work. Melinda did mention home and family issues first and then fell silent. Rather than focus in on the words being used to describe the home situation, Ms. Sykes chose to probe further, asking Melinda to expand on some of her comments. Melinda continued to be reticent, so the teacher asked, "I'm still not sure what is bothering you the most, so could you tell me what's causing you the most problems?"

Melinda paused, then shifted topics to mention her boyfriend, Randy, who had been providing much-needed emotional support for the problems at home. The 16-year-old boyfriend had been pressing Melinda for a commitment regarding their future relationship. Randy's demands and Melinda's uncertainty related to the sexual dimension of the relationship were complications that Melinda did not know how to address. Parents were not available or interested in helping her, nor did Melinda feel at all comfortable in raising such issues with them.

The teacher was able to establish that issues surrounding the boyfriend were much higher on Melinda's priority list than the family problems. Thus, the two agreed to deal, over the course of several meetings, with strategies that Melinda could use to become more assertive with her boyfriend and become more effective at problem solving. The two also discussed how information generated in the meetings would be handled and how each party had responsibilities and rights in the process of dealing with issues. Ms. Sykes felt comfortable helping Melinda, who, as a former student, had been an active member of her class. The teacher had some experience in helping students with personal problems and had even taken two counseling courses to increase her skills.

The practitioner may be faced with similar situations in which concerns are raised by the client and lead to eventual service goals. Other possibilities for issues can be shaped by the client electing to meet on an announced topic, such as thoughts of suicide, problems with studies, or any theme considered worthy of service by the practitioner. Schools concerned with problems such as drug abuse, eating disorders, or suicidal ideation have advertised the accessibility of private counseling, hoping to attract students for much-needed service. But some students will be hesitant to seek out "strangers," preferring to speak to familiar teachers.

An additional focus for sessions can come from a third party, such as a parent or school administrator, who has requested counseling for the student. As might be expected, the practitioner or student could have reservations about beginning a relationship not based on trust or mutual interest. Given the importance most practitioners place on getting a commitment to change before counseling begins, the staff member and student would need to clarify whether counseling would continue and with what goals. If, for example, a parent has referred a child for counseling, one decision to be addressed by the practitioner would be whether to pursue the referral, involve the student and the parent in some joint endeavor, or refer the parent to other service providers. In the above example, if Melinda had come unwillingly at her mother's insistence to Ms. Sykes, the teacher might not have been able to draw out information about the difficulties with the boyfriend. Rather than waste the time and energies of client and teacher, negotiation on the services of the practitioner could be conducted with the third party to define alternatives to counseling. If the parents wanted the counselor to "fix" Melinda, the teacher could opt to consult with the parents about their concerns and work to enhance their problem-solving skills. If Melinda came unwillingly but after talking with the teacher decided that she had sufficient motivation and trust to continue meeting, then Ms. Sykes could focus discussion to set goals for these future contacts.

Analysis of the Problem

The second segment of counseling will address the influences that support the presenting problem. Activities of the counselor will focus on understanding the client, conditions that contribute to problems for the client, and options available to address the problems. Again, the theoretical orientation of the practitioner can influence the strategies used to analyze the problem.

Understanding the client is the result of a complex process that involves interviewing the student, reflecting on the content and process of his/her remarks, and imposing a set of decision rules that will result in the counselor pursuing a course of action. Skills for successful interviewing have been identified by Benjamin (1981), who characterizes the interview as covering three stages (initiation, exploration, closing). Skills include questioning (open versus closed, direct versus indirect), interviewee-centered responses and leads (silence, minimal encouragers, restatement, clarification, reflection, interpretation, and explanation), interviewer-centered leads and responses (encouragement, assurance–reassurance, suggestion, advice, urging, and moralizing), and authority leads and responses (agreement–disagreement, approval–disapproval, opposition and criticism, disbelief, ridicule, contradiction, denial and rejection, scolding, threats, command, and punishment). The leads and responses can be used by the practitioner at any stage of work with the student. In an Addendum to this chapter, we provide examples of Benjamin's skills for interviewing. Understanding the child will evolve from the information gathered during initial and subsequent interviews. As the professional grows more confident in understanding the client, decision rules on a relevant course of action can be applied. Every human interchange contains choices, both in the words and signals being exchanged and in the directions taken by the participants. The practitioner operates within limitations imposed by the school system and a sense of professional ethics. The student operates within a personal set of standards and limits imposed by family and school. The professional conducts activities in the best interests of the child and system, whereas the student will work to please family, school, and personal expectations.

With all these restraints, the reader will not be surprised to hear that the best course of action in working with the student will have little to do with textbook theories and philosophies. The luxury of unlimited time for services does not exist in the public (or private) schools. Limits on staff availability, interest levels of the student and parents, and time within which to achieve gains are very real influences on the practitioner's choice of the counseling role.

Intervention Stage

The choice to work with a student on an individual basis will be influenced by the overall preferences of the professional (that person's skill and interest in working on a one-to-one basis), preferences of the student and family, and the system's flexibility to devote time on an individual basis. Within the intervention stage there will be possibilities of limited or extended services focusing on the presenting problem. The counselor can combine traditional services as outlined in Chapter 4 with guidance of the student directed at assisting in academic decision making.

One prerequisite to any intervention is frequent contact between the designated student and the school practitioner. With skill, and using the guidelines discussed in this chapter, the professional can provide a service that extends across several contacts with the student.

In addition to meeting and talking, many educators will want to include homework assignments as commonly featured in behavioral forms of counseling. The client is allowed to decide on an agreement for new behaviors, and the educator checks back to see how the commitment to change is progressing. A series of such contracts moving the student toward desired change falls within the parameters of intervention.

An example can illustrate how a teacher worked to help a student to recognize the logical consequences of his behavior (one intervention used by Adlerian counselors). The student needed several meetings to recognize his role in the problems he was experiencing. The teacher provided support for learning new perceptions and gave practice on how he could integrate these perceptions with behaviors.

TEACHER: I want you to try to notice what you are thinking and doing when I call your name in class. O.K.?
STUDENT: I think so.
TEACHER: It sounds like you're not too sure. Why don't you we try it and then get back together to discuss what you notice.

At a subsequent meeting, the teacher could continue the discussion with the student. In this case, the teacher worked to have the child learn that his behavior contributed to the consequences he had been receiving from the teacher, in this case disciplinary action.

Evaluation Stage

The success of the professional's actions will be influenced by a number of factors, including the student's motivation to cooperate with the practitioner in carrying out selected activities. In addition to the student's efforts, the time and energy devoted by the professional will play an important role influencing outcomes.

Efforts to evaluate the effectiveness of outcomes can help the professional identify actions that proved especially valuable in helping the student. Being able to learn from experiences will complement another important benefit of evaluation—being able to identify, for students, parents, and administrators, the extent to which the goals of counseling were fulfilled.

Parents, who represent important consumers of the school's services, will be very interested in being informed of what occurred over the course of individual counseling with their child. The student may or may not have kept the parents informed of the school's activities. Similarly, school administrators responsible for overall level of services may require information on the process or products of activities. Some officials will be satisfied with simple statistics defining the extent of services over a number of students, but others will request more detailed information related to a case that meets their interest (for example, when they are aware of a situation and know that the parents are interested in outcomes). Confidentiality between the practitioner and client will influence what can or will be transmitted to parents or other parties, such as administrators.

Evaluation can be conducted either informally or formally. The practitioner may use a log or other form of documentation that specifies services and descriptive information. Documentation of initial goals and the actions taken to influence the child can be examined at the end of counseling to verify the extent to which activities were delivered as planned. The issue of formative versus summative evaluation is of relevance in such considerations. Did activities get conducted within the time frame and following procedures as planned (formative evaluation)? Did changes in the student's behavior, thoughts, or affect occur as planned, as documented by observable evidence (summative evaluation)?

Professionals may be satisfied with evidence gathered from "eyeballing" the student, looking for changes in conduct or reports from key people in the student's life (parents, teachers, peers). More rigorous standards of evidence can be applied, so that the staff member has written documentation of student gains. Questionnaires or rating forms can be mailed to parents or teachers asking for feedback on recent student behavior. As with all forms of such data gathering, biasing of the reports can be expected. After all, when teachers and parents view such forms, they already know that the student has been involved in some form of school-based service. More objective forms of evidence, whether from an independent observer or from some other strategy, to document change appear needed by the entire counseling profession.

Behavioral approaches to counseling contain within them a strategy for evaluation that appears tailor-made for documenting changes. The behavioral technique involves gathering information on the presenting problem before the student receives services (labeled baseline data) and then gathering data on identically specified behaviors after the services are completed. There is, of course, the option of maintaining data gathering over the course of the counseling intervention so that information on the process of change is obtained. Chapter 4 expands on options within the evaluation stage.

IDENTIFICATION OF STUDENTS FOR INDIVIDUAL COUNSELING

Public schools, by including a counseling component within their system of services, generally have well-established policies for identifying students and referring them for counseling (Box 3.4). These procedures, however, often expose students to the counselor for services all students receive (for example, guidance on course selection or plan of study) or result from crisis-oriented concerns (for example, the school receives word that the student is having a specific difficulty that is causing others concern). Events in the student's life, at home or at school, can become public information, hastening the response of a school official or counselor. Chapter 2 contains an extensive discussion on the mechanics of the referral process.

Prevention-oriented programs similarly can be used by the school for all students (for example, drug information/prevention program) or for students considered at risk (for example, students of divorced parents, truants, students working with juvenile justice services). Formal programs will have some established procedures for funneling students toward services.

Other sources for referral will be classroom teachers, aides, and parents concerned with the actions or verbalizations of students. Within the school, word of mouth may be sufficient to link the student with the counselor, or a formal written request may be necessary to accomplish the same outcome. Parents, similarly, may contact the counselor directly for service or may need to follow a specific procedure involving written documentation and permission to effect services.

Some school districts, reflecting the economic circumstances of the

BOX 3.4. Criteria for Identifying Students for Individual Counseling

Contact with primary prevention programs
   Will all students receive exposure to information/skill-building activities? If yes, consider other criteria.

Urgency of problems
   Is student exposed to situations indicating possible harm? If yes, identify source of problems and alert support professionals and parents.

Nature of problems
   If problem is school related, gather information from student and staff to determine extent of needs and availability of resources.
   If problem is family related, gather information from student to determine scope of problem, length of concern, contact with other professionals, and establish what has been done. As necessary, initiate mandatory reporting procedures.

Who initiated contact?
   If parents, determine their involvement and planned role in counseling.
   If student, establish willingness of student to proceed. If colleagues, gather supportive information related to their concern.
   If you, contact a colleague to validate concern. Colleague could be a consultant for duration of involvement.

communities they serve, have eliminated staff counseling positions in whole or part. One strategy to remedy loss of services by some districts is to expect and train teachers to carry out limited counseling services. One district reportedly cut all counseling services at the elementary school level and trained teachers in basic communication and problem-solving skills to use with students. Prevention-oriented programs were built into the curriculum, and school psychologists were assigned crisis intervention situations.

Whatever the circumstances of the local system, counseling staff can help all school professionals to understand referral policies and identification priorities. Without such understanding and staff cooperation, the scope and impact of services will be limited.

Formal counseling services form one dimension of the counseling that goes on in schools. As we have stressed thus far in this text, many school practitioners either will have an interest in initiating counseling-like services with children or will respond affirmatively to the student requesting help. The staff member's goal can always be to prevent failure in the student's life, whether in school, the home, or the community. Too many children have been casualties of uncaring adults. School practitioners, including teachers and aides, are front-line professionals in touch with children experiencing both the everyday and occasional traumas of growing up. The professional's desire to reach out and express caring can include individual counseling for many students. As students experience trust and respect from the staff person, other students and parents soon will hear of the availability of an important resource, a school practitioner willing to extend beyond role definitions to help others.

PRACTICAL IMPLEMENTATION ISSUES

As noted above, school systems, with their budgetary restraints, will determine the extent to which counseling services exist. Priority for counseling services will reflect the political as well as economic realities of the system. Professional educators, administrators, and support service staff will have a voice in how services are selected and implemented.

Without delving into the specifics of implementation (discussed in sections of other chapters), we would note that political and economic considerations can outweigh professional preferences for "best practices" within any system. Parental influence, as many have emphasized in the literature, plays a key role in motivating systems to devote staff time and resources to counseling services. Group programs focused on widely known issues such as alcohol abuse, suicide, and teen pregnancy are visible components of service and may receive greater support from parents than will individual counseling. Given the funding levels and priorities of education, individual attention can be a service option that is difficult to sell to cost conscious administrators. Professionals, through their organizations and involvement with parent organizations, can influence the priority attached to individual approaches. Many counselors express frustration with their limited time to deliver such interventions. By using the leverage of professional expertise and influence, counselors can have a voice in the shape that a program of services takes.

School administrators at the district and building level can recognize the importance of infusing counseling-related activities across all experiences that children receive in school. Through in-service workshops and other forms of training, teachers, administrators, and support personnel can be introduced to and prepared to engage in the many forms of service that have been described in this chapter. In-class activities that emphasize the development of social skills and effective communication techniques can be part of the normal, everyday training that children receive. With a basis established for developing children's affective, behavioral, and cognitive domains, school practitioners will have access to the thoughts and feelings of children, and be able to respond as needed to the individual student. The school can become a place where trust and caring are always in display.

ADDENDUM: SKILLS FOR INTERVIEWERS

Skills that can be used in counseling cover a wide range of verbal and nonverbal techniques. As referenced above, Benjamin provides a system by which professionals can be prepared to use effective communication skills in counseling and information gathering (Box 3.5). The open–closed question distinction is basic to the interview process and can produce for a practitioner the depth of information necessary for effective decision making. Open questions allow the professional to direct the student's attention to broad dimensions of a problem, producing a response that expands beyond a simple "yes" or "no" answer. If, for example, the teacher asks Melinda, "What do you tell your parents when your boyfriend asks you to spend the night with him?" an open question has been used. Ms. Sykes's intent is to have Melinda provide commentary on a situation that will allow the teacher to have greater understanding of the dynamics of the family.

A closed question might be used, such as, "Is it true that your parents never find out that you are gone for the night?" Here the teacher is attempting to confirm previous comments by the student.

BOX 3.5. Skills for Interviewers

We support the following as helpful under many conditions:

Questions: Open versus closed

Interviewee-centered responses and leads
  Silence
  Minimal encouragers
  Restatement
  Paraphrasing/clarification
  Reflection of feelings
  Explanation

Interviewer-centered responses and leads
  Encouragement
  Assurance
  Suggestion
  Advice

The closed question can lead to either confirmation or disconfirmation, in both instances assisting the teacher in her efforts to understand the student and the presenting problem.

Benjamin's distinction between direct and indirect questions centers on the tendency of some interviewers to use a declarative statement that contains an implicit question rather than more openly raising an issue. For example, if Ms. Sykes had stated, "I wonder how your parents react when you spend the night with your boyfriend," she would be using an indirect question.

The next major cluster of skills are the interviewee-centered responses and leads. The response versus lead distinction reflects an important dimension of the practitioner–student exchange. As Bergen (1977) has noted, the communication skills of the interviewer must ensure that person's control over the exchange process. When the professional uses a lead, he/she is shaping the direction of the communication and providing an impetus that affects the process of the exchange. When the practitioner uses a response, the comments reflect the content of the previous remarks of the student. As will often happen, the professional can use the response to initiate a lead directing the student toward clarification, expansion, or a new direction in the conversation. For example:

Ms. SYKES: So when your boyfriend asks you out for the night, you generally say yes. [response] What do you do to prevent your family from finding out about your absences? [lead]

Again, the skills of the professional will have much to do with the process and products of the interview. Although some people may be uncomfortable with the notion of control, the practitioner will need to concentrate on establishing a direction to the conversation, a direction that will work to the advantage of both participants.

Interviewee-centered skills include the use of silence. Silence allows the adult to relax and wait for the student to continue talking, take the initiative in response to a comment, or elect not to respond. Most of us are uncomfortable with silence, especially when we want the student to move toward resolving a problem. But, if we rush the student through a meeting or attempt to fill in words for the student, we will only encourage frustration or signal to the student that he/she can remain relatively passive, and we will do the work for him/her.

Minimal encouragers similarly allow us to signal the student that we would like him/her to continue talking. When combined with nonverbal attending skills such as eye contact and body posture, minimal encouragers can reinforce a message that we care about the student, are interested in what he/she is saying, and would like him/her to continue talking.

Restatement and paraphrasing can be used to indicate to the student that we have heard the content of previous remarks or function to allow the student to indicate whether we are accurate in our understanding. When used judiciously, restatement or paraphrasing fits within the natural flow of the conversation and allows the counselor to confirm what has already been related. For example:

MELINDA: Yeah, they sure were fooled. I can't believe that every time that I leave late at night, they never ask where I'm going.

Ms. SYKES: You seem to be able to go out without any challenges from your parents.

MELINDA: Right. They don't seem to care at all.

Simply repeating the words of Melinda was not Ms. Sykes's intent. Indeed, mimicking the client's words is very noticeable. One reaction that practitioners report when using restatement is that the client accuses them of sounding like a psychologist! Use restatement and paraphrasing to control the conversation, responding to prior content and leading the student toward subsequent items on your agenda.

Clarification is Benjamin's word for the use of paraphrasing to simplify what the client has just said. When the student rambles on and includes content that veers off topic, the professional can restate the essence of what was said while drawing the student back on track. For example:

MELINDA: My boyfriend says that I'm being unfair to him, and maybe I am, but what else can I do? He's laying so much pressure on me and my family is bugging me and school's getting so intense, so I don't know what to do.

Ms. SYKES: You are having a tough time figuring out what to do, especially about your boyfriend. [focus on boyfriend issue]

Reflection of feelings extends the paraphrasing skill to emotions or affect. A difficult skill to implement and one that can direct the conversation to deeper levels of content than those previously discussed, reflection of feelings is a logical step when the professional wants to consider issues centering around emotions rather than thoughts (Box 3.6). Reflection, because the process evokes emotions, requires both the establishment of trust with the student and the skill to deal with the emotions once they are confirmed and become part of the counseling's agenda. In our ongoing saga, when Melinda begins

BOX 3.6. Practicing Reflecting Feelings

GOALS

1. To provide opportunity to practice reflecting feelings.
2. To stimulate the recognition of expressed feelings.
3. To stimulate the use of reflecting feeling statements.
4. To provide feedback on the use of the skill.

DIRECTIONS

Practice Alone

1. For the following two statements, write a single "feeling word" ("tag word") that concretely labels the speaker's feelings. No single word is correct. Several words will have the same effect. This exercise is intended to sharpen your hearing of words expressing feelings.

Example: "Gee, I don't know if I should. I'm worried that my mother won't like it. I'd hate for her to find out."

Tag word: _____ [worried]

Example A: "I just love pets. I wish I had even more. We have a beautiful Siamese cat. She's really fun."

Tag word: _____

Example B: "I'm worried about my blood pressure. I hope the readings are not too high."

Tag word: _____

2. For the following, write a response that accurately reflects the expressed feelings.

Example C: "Gee, I feel better. I was just moping along feeling sorry for myself. Thanks for listening."

Response: _____
_____
_____

Example D: "I'm so nervous about my speech. I hope I can remember it."

Response: _____
_____
_____

Example E: "Sometimes I hate giving grades. It's so hard to be objective. I just wish teachers didn't have to give grades. It spoils the fun of teaching."

Response: _____
_____
_____

(continued)

BOX 3.6. (*Continued*)

Practice with Feedback

1. In groups of three, assign roles (observer, speaker, listener). Speaker tells a personal story that makes reference to feelings. Listener practices reflecting feelings. Observer makes note of reflections. Reactions are shared; then roles are rotated.

2. In a small group, one person relates a story that contains references to feelings, a second person practices reflecting feelings, and other members observe and give feedback to the person practicing. When giving feedback, be sure it is positive. Continue until all members have a chance to reflect feelings and receive feedback.

3. In a large group, form inner (vocal participants) and outer circles (silent observers). Inner circle members conduct a discussion that allows all to practice reflecting feelings. Topics for discussion might be "My biggest disappointment" or "My most embarrassing moment." Observers use the *Reflecting Feelings Form* to tally observations and then provide feedback followed by discussion. Inner and outer circle members then switch roles.

REFLECTING FEELINGS FORM

Name of person being observed:

Your name: _____

Directions: Jot down a short notation or paraphrase of the reflecting responses that the target person makes. Note whether the reflection was accurate and whether it contains a concrete feeling or tag word. Jot down the tag word.

Reflection	Accurate?	Tag word
1.		
2.		
3.		
4.		
5.		
6.		
7.		

Other observations

to relate how she feels about some of the family problems and relations with the boyfriend, the teacher can choose to delve into the tone and meaning of the comments to reveal affect.

Reflection of feelings represents the beginning of the practitioner's efforts to work on emotions. For example:

MELINDA: I just don't understand why he can't leave me alone. I tell him what he seems to want to hear, and yet he keeps on bugging me.

Ms. SYKES: You feel frustrated when he doesn't seem to understand.

Ms. Sykes's comment qualifies as a paraphrase of the surface of Melinda's message and focuses attention on the feeling that she is experiencing as she reports both past events and reactions outside the context of counseling.

Interpretation is another variant of paraphrasing, but one that introduces consideration of the adult's or student's frame of reference. As Benjamin notes, the school practitioner can choose either dimension of reference when interpreting remarks of the student. For example:

MELINDA: Just because I'm the oldest, my parents expect me to take more responsibilities than my brothers and sister. I'm expected to step into all the fights so that my parents don't have to be bothered.

Ms. SYKES: You don't like being the oldest, especially with your parents' expectations.

The teacher deals with the content using a paraphrase yet takes Melinda's perspective, not the parents', in reflecting on the events being described. The teacher's frame of reference could be introduced if she stated:

Ms. SYKES: I was the oldest, too, and I can understand the frustration you must be feeling.

Johnson (1986) has stressed that interpretation of client comments can interfere with progress in counseling. By imposing one or more levels of interpretation on remarks, the practitioner can distract the client from efforts to reflect on experiences of past events. The adult can introduce too much of himself/herself into the conversation, intruding into the student's efforts to make sense of thoughts or emotions. By directing the student's attention toward our own perceptions or reactions, we take away some of the responsibility of the client to interpret what has transpired.

Explanation as a separate skill can involve evaluation but, at its simplest, represents a logical statement of events or circumstances. The adult can elect to state to the client an explanation that deals with orientation to the situation, behavior, causes, or the interviewer's position.

Orientation to the situation would include the professional's remarks about what the student could expect during the counseling sessions. For example, Ms. Sykes could say, "We will be spending time just talking about what's on your mind. What we talk about will stay between the two of us."

Explanation of behavior is similarly straightforward. Ms. Sykes, at an early stage of working with Melinda, might say, "We are meeting today in part because of the concerns of your English teacher, who came to me when you said you wanted to talk to someone about problems at home." The comment by the teacher ensured that Melinda would not misunderstand either the actions or intentions of her comments.

Explanation of causes allows the professional to comment on remarks by the client, especially those that underline some of the frustrations being reported by the client. For example:

MELINDA: I just don't know why I can't confront my boyfriend.

Ms. SYKES: Because you have a lot of tension in your life and no idea what to do to solve a problem, I can see why you would have a hard time confronting the one person who really cares about you.

Explanation of causes lets the practitioner make sense of portions of what the client has reported. Such statements should be used with caution to avoid applying an interpretation of events that is off target. The client, for example, could be commenting selectively on past situations, thus presenting an inaccurate picture of what has occurred. By leaping into an explanation based on faulty information, the professional could both solidify the distortion as fact and encourage the client to introduce additional distortions to the exchange.

Explanation of the interviewer's position is the professional's effort to state what he/she believes about portions of the conversation's content. When the adult takes a stand on an issue, the explanation serves the purpose of informing the client about the content and boundaries of that stand. For example, in dealing with the notion of confidentiality during sessions, Ms. Sykes could have remarked to Melinda as follows:

Ms. SYKES: We can discuss anything you would like during our meetings. I want you to realize that I cannot keep everything between us confidential. If you have been abused or have intentions of hurting yourself or others, I must contact agencies outside of the school. Our state has a law that says that when a person is abused physically or sexually, a counselor must report the circumstances to the Department of Human Services. [Goes on to deal with additional issues and limitations.]

The most important advice to all school practitioners working with students is to remain aware of both the content and tone of the client's message. Without consistent awareness of the student, the most powerful of the interviewee-centered skills will be of little use. The next set of skills, though useful during many counseling activities, are more often seen in other attempts to deal with students. A teacher, administrator, or support professional may use any of the following during noncounseling activities, such as advising, consulting, leading classroom academic activities, or even disciplining students.

Interviewer-centered leads and responses comprise the next set of skills identified by Benjamin. Encouragement of the client is a prerequisite to all others, in that we must work to have the client talk with us before any other actions on our part. Encouragement is a verbal and nonverbal process involving all the signals that we send to the client to reinforce communication. Johnson (1986) emphasizes that our verbal and nonverbal signals must be congruent for maximum effectiveness. We can't, for instance, tell the student we are interested in what he/she is saying when we are working hard to stifle a yawn!

Assurance and reassurance are actions we take to indicate our support of or belief in the client. As we work to establish trust, we must signal that we are hearing the descriptions of problems and can empathize with the client's efforts to deal with situations. We can function additionally to motivate the client to try out new behaviors or to apply existing skills in new situations.

For example, when Melinda discussed boyfriend problems, the teacher noticed that Melinda had been successful in confronting the boyfriend on other issues in the past yet was hesitant to behave similarly now. Ms. Sykes stated, "I'm confident that you can bring out your concerns about sex. You understand the risks involved and really care about how these conflicts are affecting your relationship." The teacher's comments are not intended to convince the student of something she is incapable of doing but rather function to boost her confidence to address a concern that has been taking up much of her time in figuring out what to do. Indeed, the teacher's comments can function to strip away distortions that may be influencing the decision-making capabilities of the student.

Suggestion is a restricted form of advice in which the professional raises the possibility of certain courses of action or thought. As with all forms of suggestions, the practitioner must balance several considerations: wanting to guide the client without fostering dependence; wanting to wait for the client to initiate suggestions without frustration influencing commitment to the counseling process; and wanting the client to initiate a search for alternatives without imposing closure.

In our instance, Ms. Sykes, on observing Melinda's difficulty in deciding how to begin her planned confrontation with the boyfriend, said:

Ms. SYKES: The hardest part of this type of situation is what to say first.

MELINDA: But what can I say? I've thought this over a hundred times and still don't know what to do.

Ms. SYKES: I was thinking that you could start just by describing how frustrated you have been about this whole situation and how thinking about this has affected school and getting along with your family. How does that sound?

The teacher wants to leave plenty of opportunity for Melinda to choose her own course of action. After all, the teacher has no idea what the boyfriend thinks, feels, or is capable of doing, having access only to Melinda's descriptions of her perceptions of the boyfriend.

A more forceful technique would involve giving advice to the client. Almost every author of a text on counseling has commented on the value of advice within the context of helping. More often than not, advice giving is discouraged. Most writers believe that advice giving takes away the client's responsibility for selecting a course of action. At best, advice can be based on a misreading of the client and at worst can promote passivity and dependence in the client. There are plenty of adults in the child's life already more than willing to provide advice!

At the level of common sense, we realize that advice giving need not be so complicated. The client is free to reject any and all comments on our part. Life is full of people giving advice, some good and some bad. An important consideration for the practitioner, however, involves professional responsibility for the consequences of the comments that are made to the client. When advice is given, the practitioner must be sensitive to the client's capabilities for successfully achieving what has been proposed. The need for follow-up of the student is heightened. The position taken by most authors is that when a counselor gives advice, he/she must also allow flexibility as to what is being proposed and be sure that the client recognizes that he/she has the freedom to accept or reject any suggestion. Urging the client to adopt a behavior allows the professional to motivate the student while maintaining a focus on who is responsible for initiating that behavior. The motivational component of urging is at the center of what is being suggested by the practitioner. In other words, the client and professional agree on what could be done, yet the student appears unwilling or unsure about what to do. The goal of urging is to direct the student's attention toward what has been or could be planned. For example:

Ms. SYKES: I thought that you had decided to confront your boyfriend this weekend. You were so committed to resolving your problem that I am surprised that you didn't even bring it up.

MELINDA: Well, I thought I was ready to talk to him, but when I saw him, I just couldn't say anything. I felt that I was being so unfair to him.

Ms. SYKES: Of course you can tell him what you think and feel. We have talked about the many times he has hassled you and caused you pain. I think you are ready to deal with him, and I'm here to help you prepare for what you're going to do. How about doing some more role playing and see how you could set up the conversation so that he will listen to you.

MELINDA: O.K. I guess I'm ready to finish this whole thing, too.

Moralizing has proven controversial in the counseling literature, with most writers lining up in opposition to its use. Benjamin (1981) notes that moralizing extends beyond urging or persuading to include reference to conscience or morals. Although he recognizes that moralizing can have a positive impact on the client, Benjamin says that the professional must be prepared for a more likely response—resistance or displeasure on the part of the client. Johnson (1986) seconds Benjamin's caution and urges avoidance of moralizing in any situation within which we hope to maintain client trust and participation.

For example, in our case involving Melinda, the teacher could have stated, "You realize that you owe your parents an explanation for what you have been doing. After all, you are a minor and should not be engaging in sex, and they are responsible for you." Melinda would be unusual indeed if she did not react negatively to the professional's remarks. Whether she chose to not say anything or make a remark at that time, Melinda was faced with deciding whether she could trust further in the teacher. Johnson's suggestion is to emphasize paraphrasing and understanding of the client rather than to adopt a moralizing stand. Your efforts are more than likely to be rewarded with the former position.

The final cluster of skills are authority leads and responses. Benjamin classifies these skills as extending beyond the boundaries of most counseling situations. Counseling typically allows for a focus on the interviewee but can extend under select conditions to be interviewer focused. Authority leads and responses, as defined, would involve a professional who is committed to a particular course of action with the client and is willing to apply pressure on the client to accept certain identified services. Benjamin expresses discomfort with the position, in that it involves a practitioner imposing actions that the client might not have expressed an interest in considering. Benjamin does describe what a counselor could do if he/she subscribes to a philosophy that justifies such actions.

Rather than dwell on the details of each approach under this heading, we will briefly define the options (Benjamin, 1981):

1. Agreement–disagreement: The adult can express an opinion as to whether the client's decisions or ideas are right or wrong.
2. Approval–disapproval: Similar to the above, but with an opinion as to whether an action or idea is good or bad.
3. Opposition and criticism: Unambiguously expressing opposition to a course of action or unambiguously expressing displeasure with the client's conduct or plans.
4. Disbelief: Assuming that the client's perceptions are distorted and challenging the client to reflect on what has been presented as accurate. The intent is to get the client to evaluate the situation more logically.
5. Ridicule: Using condescension to underline disbelief of a client's remarks. The intent is to illustrate the absurdity of the client's words.

Additional techniques involve the use of contradiction and a more extreme strategy of denial and rejection. Only the most authoritarian of counselors would even consider such remarks, yet many readers will recognize that in school-based services, such comments are heard by some students. Services providers would do well to heed the words of Benjamin, who encourages us to use "the light touch of humor which stems from empathic listening and which reflects a positive outlook on life" (p. 159). Laughing with the client is to be preferred to any of the authority leads and responses.

4

Practical Issues of Individual Counseling

As was seen in the previous chapter, the professional who chooses to work individually with a student faces a number of restrictions on activities. Even given these restrictions, however, the professional will elect the individual counseling approach when students' needs fit within a number of characteristics. The student who needs immediate attention, who does not work well in a group context, or who is unwilling to reveal information with other persons present might motivate the professional to choose one-on-one sessions. Although counseling can begin with intensive individual contact, the option always remains for switching to a group context as appropriate. Group counseling alternatives are considered in the next two chapters.

The current chapter presents practical information with case illustrations on major issues within individual counseling. Specific techniques that have proven useful are defined. Strategies that can be used to deal with some of the more difficult problems within a school, such as truancy, vandalism, and aggression, are considered.

SESSION-BY-SESSION POINTS

In Chapter 3, the process of counseling was considered to include at least four major steps: problem identification, analysis, intervention, and evaluation. Equally important issues for the counselor to address are skills in establishing rapport with the student and problem setting.

Skills in Establishing Rapport

For the counselor to establish a helping relationship with the client, trust between the two must be established. The student, who is expected to describe thoughts and feelings for counseling to be effective, must believe that he/she is working in a climate that contains trust, acceptance, and open communication (George & Cristiani, 1986). Trust, as many writers have argued, is a prerequisite for the counseling relationship. A student's motivation to enter counseling is at best fragile and must be nurtured for trust to develop. Whatever the orientation of the counselor, whatever philosophy or model is followed, trust is essential before counseling can proceed (see Box 4.1).

The notion of acceptance follows in line with trust. Carl Rogers (1951) has written about the importance of acceptance, especially in regard to the gains that a client can experience. Rogers has argued that trust along with genuineness and acceptance will lead the client to better understand himself/herself. With more understanding, the client can become more acceptant of others and better able to cope with problems in functioning.

Barriers to communication can impede the establishment of trust and acceptance. As discussed in the last chapter, there are a number of communication techniques that range from interviewee-centered to interviewer-centered approaches. The skills can, under certain conditions, enhance progress toward resolution of problems but in

---

BOX 4.1. Establishing and Enhancing Rapport

Issues in establishing rapport
    Trust between the student and practitioner
    Student's motivation to enter counseling
    Acceptance of the student's needs
    Genuineness of student's concern and your willingness
        to become involved

Strategies to enhance rapport
    Nonverbal cues to the student
        Interested facial expression
        Relaxed posture
        Eye contact
        Open welcoming gestures
        Listening

    Verbal cues to the student
        Soft tone of voice
        Relaxed pacing of conversation
        Expression of empathy
        Focus on student's concerns

---

other situations can indeed function as barriers. Gordon (1974) has argued that giving advice, offering solutions, moralizing and preaching, analyzing and diagnosing, judging or criticizing, praising and agreeing, and reassuring can all impede the effect of communication. Such verbal behaviors, widely practiced among all human beings, tend to distract the client from the essence of change. The client's attention must be directed to maintain personal responsibility for behavior and a commitment to change.

The counselor, to establish trust, acceptance, and effective communication, must constantly monitor what is being communicated verbally and nonverbally and be sensitive to potential impact on the student. Johnson (1986) has stressed the importance of nonverbal cues to alert the client to the caring and respect the counselor has for the child. Johnson argues that a soft tone of voice, an interested facial expression, a relaxed posture, eye contact, and open welcoming gestures are all essentials to establishing contact. Rapport between the two parties is the outcome of the successful establishment of trust and acceptance. As the student becomes more relaxed, he/she will tend to reveal deeper levels of thoughts or feelings to the professional. These thoughts and feelings can be regarded by the practitioner as the focus of counseling efforts or can be taken as a stimulus to probe even more deeply into perceptions and emotions.

For example, a classroom teacher may be approached by a student to discuss progress on an assignment. The student, who has had many opportunities to see the teacher interact with others, might take the opportunity to mention some problems completing the assignment at home. The student could be attempting to discover whether the teacher will "pick up" on the reference, perhaps questioning what was creating an interference with progress. Although little may be resolved at the initial contact, the teacher can follow up on the student's work to see if problems at home are still issues for the child. As time passes and the two parties explore how the other person is thinking or feeling, trust can build, leading to discussions of deeper levels of emotion. A teacher with good skills of reflecting feelings can increase the likelihood that emotions will be brought to the surface and discussed.

Other writers have introduced the term empathy, defined as "the ability to tune in to the client's feelings and to be able to see the client's world as it truly seems to the client" (George & Cristiani, 1986, p. 154). Empathy is a concept denoting both the attitude and the affect expressed by the practitioner as the problem being presented is addressed. Without empathy, many writers would argue, the counselor will be limited in terms of potential impact on the client.

Problem Setting

Donald Schon (1983) has argued that the concept of problem setting must be considered prior to engaging in professional service, even before problem identification, our first listed stage of counseling (Box 4.2). He notes the confusion of real-world circumstances within which we experience problems. Often there is no clear-cut single problem that we can confront nor, seemingly, a clear-cut direction to resolve our difficulties. He recognizes that "when we set the problem, we select what we will treat as the 'things' of the situation, we set the boundaries of our attention to it, and we impose on it the coherence which allows us to say what is wrong and in what directions the situation needs to be changed" (Schon, 1983, p. 40). Problem setting is, thus, the process by which we determine how we will view difficulties confronting the student. Until we have focused all our attention and the student's attention on specific behaviors, thoughts, or emotions, we cannot begin to define the limits of the problem.

The idea behind problem setting is that as professionals, school practitioners will work with the client to establish the dimensions of what will be addressed within the confines of professional service. The notion of a contract between the two parties is similar, but problem setting refers to a much deeper level of analysis of the problem situation. As the student relates thoughts, behaviors, and feelings to the professional, that person will reflect on what is being communicated and place it within the context of what is known about child development, family issues, school policies, and other relevant concerns. The communication techniques used by the professional will direct the student's attention as the practitioner places all that is being discussed within a form that is understandable to both parties.

BOX 4.2. Problem Setting

The process by which we determine how we will view difficulties confronting the student. Points to consider:

1. Not everything perceived by the student as a problem will be seen as a problem by us. *Action:* Probe student's thinking to discover the criteria applied to define a behavior or event as a problem.
2. Not everything the school practitioner perceives as a problem will be seen by the student as a problem. *Action:* Alert the student to your thinking. Allow student to challenge your assumptions and evaluations. Be open to compromise on the steps taken to identify the problem. Point out logical consequences of the student's and your current behaviors.
3. The priority during problem setting is to determine the boundaries of the student's awareness of thought processes and the world around him/her. *Action:* Proceed deliberately to understand the student's perspective relevant to the presenting problem. Don't rush into goal setting.

Allen Ivey (1983) has described the technique of reflecting meaning, which might prove effective at this stage of counseling. In defining the skill of reflection of meaning, Ivey proposes that the practitioner determine just what meaning the content of the client's comments has for that person. There are three aspects to determining the meaning of content: the cognitive, the behavioral, and the affective. The cognitive aspect accounts for the attitudes and thoughts surrounding the content. What importance does the material have to the client? The behavioral aspect alludes to past actions and the planned actions of the client. Of greatest importance is the affective dimension, the feelings that the client has about the content. Using communication skills discussed in earlier sections, the school practitioner attempts to reflect accurately the meaning of what is being said.

For example, open questions can be used to uncover the cognitive underpinnings of a statement.

STUDENT: I think I'd better drop your course.
TEACHER: What seems to be the problem?

Paraphrases are also helpful in reflecting back content to the client.

TEACHER: It seems that your job is taking so much time that you don't have a chance to study.

To address affect (and display empathy), the practitioner can reflect feelings.

STUDENT: I really don't want to drop the class. I feel like a quitter.
TEACHER: It sounds as though this is hard for you.

Schon's priority in discussing problem setting is to alert professionals to the need to monitor more effectively their thoughts while working with students. In other words, school practitioners need to be more in tune with what is going on in their own heads as the student provides information. The professional needs to reflect on options for communicating with the student as well as on the best strategy for pursuing additional information. Schon goes on to argue that one way to be successful as a reflective practitioner is to encourage the client, by example, to relate openly information about a situation and be willing to challenge the professional as that person leads the student toward problem solving.

For example, in one rural district, the counselor was approached by a student, Amy, who wanted a note to the teacher excusing her from classes that she had missed for 3 days in a row. The counselor, Mr.

Abrams, took the opportunity of Amy's approaching him to sit down with her and to discuss what was on her mind while she was at school. Amy, who had worked with Mr. Abrams previously, needed little stimulation to discuss a number of things that were bothering her. Difficulties with peers, with teachers, siblings, and parents all seemed of equal importance as she began to discuss what was bothering her. Mr. Abrams chose to let her talk rather than to ask many questions, but before too long he began to notice that Amy's comments kept returning to peer issues. With the use of a few open questions ("What happens next?" "What did you do then?"), Mr. Abrams began to see a definite pattern in how Amy perceived classmates. Amy, through the example she provided, indicated that she set pretty high standards for what friends should and should not do to her. When a friend violated these standards, Amy's response was typically to be very upset and to shun her peers. With a clearer idea of how Amy engaged in problem setting, Mr. Abrams reached a choice point of his own: Should he work further with Amy to deal with what she perceived as a difficulty, or should he simply listen and indicate general support and try to get Amy back into class?

Such choices exist all the time in the schools. School practitioners trying to balance available time and energy may elect to be a "shoulder to cry on" and work hard to keep students academically engaged. In the above situation, Mr. Abrams decided that Amy did need someone who was a good listener, not someone who wanted to come in and help her be more effective solving her own problems. Mr. Abrams also knew that Amy would be available for future contact if she preferred to wait to learn new skills for dealing with peers.

An additional consideration in problem setting involves limitations on the professional's response. What issues or presenting problems will motivate the professional to intervene? As with Amy, the counselor may be looking for specific signals of how a student deals with problem circumstances. An additional consideration might be the impact of the student's behavior on others. When other teachers are concerned, the practitioner may be more likely than otherwise to intervene.

Problem Identification

As noted in the last chapter, when the practitioner and client agree on the focus of counseling, problem identification has been initiated. Often in a school setting, staff members will have some background information on the students, at times gathered from direct observation and at others from school records. With existing referral mechanisms within the school building, counselors and other support professionals may have already taken the opportunity to chat with teachers, administrators, or other staff members about the student who has asked to meet to discuss a problem. Problem identification will center on establishing a clear idea on the course that counseling will take. A logical outcome of problem identification will be the professional and the student agreeing on what goals can be achieved for the student. Skills used by the professional during problem identification include those covered in the Chapter 3 Addendum (see Box 4.3).

The problem identification meeting may last more than one session. As many school people are aware, students may approach us with seeming motivation to talk about concerns but, when pressed to communicate, have a great deal of difficulty opening up. The student may need several attempts at communicating before he/she has sufficient trust to relate difficulties.

Similarly, the staff member may use one or more sessions to focus the attention of the student on problems occurring in his/her life. Some approaches to counseling, such as the behavioral, will actually assign the student homework so that the student comes back to a

---

BOX 4.3. Tips on Problem Identification

1. Organize available background information on the student.
   - Review files and information from student, classmates, staff, parents.
   - Consider previous documentation, if any, of counseling assistance.

2. Solicit student's description of concerns/problems.
   - Focus on content of student's comments.
   - Recognize affect underlying content.
   - Reflect/check out affect.
   - Request elaboration and validation of information during each contact.
   - Ask student to prioritize needs/preferences.

3. Determine your willingness and availability to be of assistance.
   - Assess time and energy needed to help student.
   - Evaluate your expertise in counseling students with the identified problem.
   - Identify resources to help as needed.

4. Build bridges to future contact.
   - Refer to other services (see Boxes 2.1 and 2.2) if your choose not to counsel.
   - Confirm nature of your willingness to be involved.
   - Assign student responsibility for gathering any information necessary to assist in goal setting.
   - Plan future meetings.

---

second session having acquired specific information on frequency of problem behaviors.

Problem identification will involve students talking about a range of issues affecting them in their lives. Topics to be addressed can include how the student is dealing with school assignments, how the student is relating to peers, and how things are going at home. Such conversation leads can be pursued with the student by the professional unless the client takes the lead and presents a problem to be discussed.

Many times, students will have a suitcase full of problems that are on their mind at any one time. During problem identification, the professional can spend the time sorting through bits and pieces of information about a child, trying to make sense about what is occurring in that child's life, and establish some rank ordering of the seeming importance of these difficulties. The student will, of course, play an important role and attach priorities to which problems should be addressed in which sequence.

Many school professionals realize that the intensity of the presenting problem will play an important role in the emphasis that is assigned to working with the student. As a result, some professionals consider the initial contact with the student as more of an open-ended interview that can allow the professional to make preliminary decisions about presenting problems. Even if there is no short preliminary meeting, the problem identification stage can shift focus back and forth between issues such as client–counselor responsibility, presenting problems and their prioritization, and potential goals for working with the student. The professional approaches the client with at least one objective in mind: to spend some time exploring how the student perceives his/her circumstances and, by so doing, highlighting possible problems shading those perceptions.

One recommended outcome of problem identification is having the client leave the session confident that something can be done to address his/her concerns. In essence, a bridge can be constructed between the present, in which the student has concerns, and the future, in which the two parties will be working on those concerns. When those concerns, however, border on the capacity of the professional to be effective, alternatives can be considered by which the student can receive other services.

The concern being expressed here is when to refer the student to other appropriate services. Educators may be mandatory reporters of certain events and not expected to delve into the circumstances until outside agencies make their investigations. When to refer can center on the practitioner's competencies, available time and energies, and the seriousness of the presenting problem. The school building itself may have a crisis team or office available to deal with pressing problems that extend beyond the scope of school-based services. George and Cristiani (1986, pp. 139–140) have provided a helpful list of when the professional should consider referring the client for other services. The authors state that referral should occur when:

1. The client presents a problem that is beyond your level of competency.
2. When you feel that personality differences between you and the client cannot be resolved or will interfere with the counseling process.
3. When the client is a personal friend or relative, and the concern is going to require an ongoing relationship.
4. When the client is reluctant to discuss this problem with you for some reason.
5. When, after several sessions, you do not feel your relationship with the client is effective.

Referring the student to an available counselor in the building can be an easy alternative in some schools. Other schools will have only one counselor, and the referral, when appropriate, may be to an outside mental health agency. Complications to such referrals include fees for services, students' willingness to go to nonschool services, and parental support for nonschool help. George and Cristiani's final recommendation about referral is that the practitioner specify a particular person in the referred agency so that the student's parents have a clear idea of whom to contact.

Problem identification, thus, is a complex process of encouraging the students to talk, making sense and interpretations of their comments, and motivating them to work within the context of individual counseling. The better the practitioner is as a listener, the more able that person will be to absorb the information being transmitted by the student. An example of a successful problem identification meeting comes from a junior high school in which the school psychologist, Ms. Irons, has received notice that James is upset and refuses to leave his literature class.

Ms. Irons, with an established procedure of backing up teachers, went to the literature class to see what she could do to help. James had been disciplined earlier in that class and argued quite loudly that he was being treated unfairly. With some encouragement from the psychologist and teacher, James did walk with Ms. Irons to her office.

After covering the territory of the difficulty in class, Ms. Irons asked James how things were going for him in general at school. For the next 20 minutes, all Ms. Irons heard was a litany of complaints about teachers and classmates being unfair to him. Indeed, Ms. Irons was impressed by James's memory: he was able to recall words and actions of other people that had occurred over the past several weeks. The theme of the conversation was thus easy to identify, but how did James see the difficulties that he was encountering?

James did show some insight into the common thread connecting all his difficulties in school. He had talked with one teacher who taught his industrial arts class about some of his troubles in getting along with others. His parents were threatening to punish him if he didn't get along better at school.

Ms. Irons offered her support for working on his problem of getting along and indicated that she was running a small group of other students in the school to talk about similar issues. James denied that he had a big problem but also indicated he did not want other people to know about his inability to deal with others. Ms. Irons was aware of some of James's history of having difficulty getting along with classmates. To her surprise, James indicated that he would be willing to talk with her to deal with some of his difficulties.

After getting a commitment, Ms. Irons reviewed, using the technique of paraphrasing, several of the episodes that James had related around the issue of problems with peers and teachers. When James confirmed that these episodes had occurred and were troubling him, Ms. Irons pursued his comment by asking him which group caused the most problems for him—adults or peers. James was much more concerned about the reactions of peers than adults but did indicate an awareness that he needed to get along with teachers and administrators at school if he wanted to graduate.

With this confirmation of the priorities of his concerns, Ms. Irons asked James to come back 2 days from then with a listing of what had occurred in that 48-hour period in terms of his interactions with others. James asked for a little help on what he should be listing, so Ms. Irons said, "What I want you to do is to act as you would normally act, but when you do find yourself feeling frustrated or getting into conflicts with others, I want you to write down everything that you can remember as soon as you leave the situation." She showed him an example of what another student had done in a previous year. The example had been modified so that the student who had completed the form was not identified, nor were other persons mentioned in the report. James expressed some discomfort about writing down something for the psychologist to see, but Ms. Irons soon figured out that he was worried that she might evaluate his writing skills. Promising not to take note of misspellings or grammar, the psychologist encouraged James to try out the system for at least 2 days and get back to her. At that point, recognizing that there would be at least one more visit around James's concerns, Ms. Irons talked a little bit more about what he could expect of her during any meetings and what she would expect of him in terms of openness and commitment to the counseling process. She reflected that what went on between them would stay within her office and because of that he should feel free to talk about his thoughts and feelings even when he was a little afraid to do so. James had no reaction to her comment at that time, but Ms. Irons was impressed that he did appear serious about trying out her suggested method of noting problem encounters with classmates and adults. The problem identification stage was initiated for both parties and would lead directly to the issues of the next stage of the counseling process, that of analysis.

Problem Analysis of Content

Making sense of all that the student has said in the early stages of counseling can challenge the most effective practitioner. The professional is always faced with the choice of dealing strictly with the content of what has occurred within counseling sessions, comparing such content to what is known about the student outside of that setting, and weighing all the facts against school policies and priorities. For example, a professional may be quite confident that what a student has related is accurate and sufficient for planning sessions. On the other hand, the staff member may have acquired quite a bit of information about the student in other settings. The student may have established a reputation for honesty or dishonesty, may have been seen in the counseling office or the principal's office in the past, or may have signaled nonverbally that much was not being said. The final possibility, that of weighing school district policies and priorities, is always important. As noted earlier, the professional at times will have no difficulty electing to offer individual counseling but at other times may be aware of group settings more appropriate to dealing with the student's needs. A final consideration might be that the practitioner is aware that neither the administration nor the parents would support the individual counseling option.

Assuming that the counselor elects to continue with the student, analysis of content becomes more relevant (Box 4.4). Problem identification will at best provide the professional with a clear idea of which problems are occurring in a student's life and which problem is considered of greatest importance by the student. Analysis begins

BOX 4.4. Problem Analysis and Planning

1. Review all information relevant to understanding the presenting problem.
2. Direct student's attention to provide details on thoughts, feelings, and behaviors related to problem.
3. Emphasize your interest in and support of the student.
4. Keep student involved and motivated by expressing your thoughts and reactions to what is being said (apply skills described in Chapter 3 Addendum).
5. Insure that problem-solving strategies produce information needed for development of intervention tactics.
6. Develop specific actions to be taken, agree on who will be responsible and the time frame for actions, and discuss monitoring and evaluation strategies.

with the presenting problem and serves as the vehicle within which the professional works to develop an intervention plan.

Successful analysis always involves some risk taking by both parties. The professional, using effective communication skills, will be directing the student's attention to provide content of thoughts, behaviors, and emotions and can quickly increase intensity of sessions to higher and higher levels. Professionals are always concerned not only about how to maintain structure and direction on the content of the sessions but also about providing students with a sense of accomplishment and motivation to maintain their attention to deal with their problems. Educators are well aware of children who leave counseling more distraught than when they came in. Maintaining control over strong negative emotions can prove to be very difficult if not impossible on occasion. Analysis can serve to bring negative emotions and thoughts closer and closer to the surface because the intent of analysis is to generate information that will assist both parties to better understand the past and the present so that future needs can be addressed. By reflecting the feelings of the client, the practitioner helps the student to understand his/her feelings.

Problem solving rests at the heart of what actually goes on during analysis. The situation that the student describes is broken down into its component parts so that both parties can determine what needs to be done in terms of client understanding, planning, and action.

At least three related models can be considered to analyze client difficulties. Stewart, Winborn, Johnson, Burks, and Engelkes (1978, p. 192) provide one model for dealing with client decision making:

1. Identify the problem. This step should include answers to problems such as: What is the problem? What prevents a solu-

tion? When and under what circumstances does the problem occur?

2. Identification of values. During this phase the client's values are examined so that the solution will be consistent with the client's values and long-range goals.
3. Identify alternatives. A list of possible alternatives is formulated.
4. Examine alternatives. At this stage the advantages and disadvantages of each proposal are weighed, based on factual information such as amount of time and money involved.
5. Make a tentative decision.

As Stewart et al. (1978) note, analysis of the situation can be accomplished by a series of questions (open as well as closed), brainstorming, and elimination of alternatives until a single course of action is determined. Krumboltz (1966, p. 156) proposes a very similar model for problem solving and decision making:

1. Generating a list of all possible courses of action.
2. Gathering relevant information about each feasible alternative course of action.
3. Estimating the probability of success in each alternative on the basis of the experience of others and projection of current needs.
4. Considering the personal values that may be enhanced or diminished under each course of action.
5. Deliberating and weighing the facts, probable outcomes, and values for each alternative.
6. Eliminating from consideration least favorable courses of action.
7. Formulating a tentative plan of action subject to new developments and opportunities.
8. Generalizing the decision-making process to future problems.

Decision making and problem solving can be accomplished using Egan's (1975) approach. The Egan model includes the following elements: (1) Identify and clarify the problem. The educator, by using effective communication skills, will direct the client's attention to difficulties being experienced, guiding the conversation so that specificity is accomplished. (2) Establish priorities in choosing problems for attention. Clients are directed to decide which problems to tackle using specific criteria that Egan defines (problems directly under client's control, crisis situations, a problem that is easily handled, a problem that when solved will bring about some improvement, and moves from lesser to greater severity). (3) Establish workable goals. Help the student to define what can feasibly be achieved in a specific time frame. (4) Take a census of available means for reaching the goal. Use a force field analysis by which the student can list restraining and facilitating forces relevant to attaining the goal. (5) Choose the means that will most effectively achieve established goals. Means may involve client action or client manipulation of others. (6) Establish criteria for the effectiveness of action programs. Help the student while setting realistic expectations to define criteria by which success can be judged.

All activities during the analysis stage will lead the professional and client to agreement on a specific course of action. Planning for action must precede the intervention stage, to be discussed later.

In our example above, Ms. Irons worked with James to make greater sense of some of the difficulties he was having in his life. As noted earlier, problems with peers quickly became the focus of the discussions with the client. The psychologist spent more than an hour getting examples of how James had dealt with peer situations in the past, quickly coming to the conclusion that James had a weak grasp of some important social skills. Ms. Irons was aware that James's skills were not much better with adults, yet recognized that James would be more motivated initially to deal with peer-addressed issues.

The psychologist spent some time helping James to think through the past encounters, trying to identify what he could have done differently so that he would have felt more successful with peers. James seemed quite aware of how his actions and words had contaminated past encounters. He had plenty of models from among his classmates who were socially successful. However, James lacked the confidence to initiate encounters that he saw the successful peers initiating.

James indicated that he was very motivated to begin work, so the psychologist spent a half hour reviewing the steps of problem solving as applied to James's difficulties. The psychologist and student agreed that James's actions were directly related to the difficulties he was experiencing. Second, the two agreed that a priority for their future encounters would be discussing how his thoughts, actions, and words could be modified to improve his social success. Third, the two agreed on a time frame of one academic semester within which James would take more and more responsibility with peers for initiating positive encounters. The skills related to these increasingly intensive encounters were not spelled out in detail during this initial meeting.

Next, the two listed the social skills that James already had that would contribute to his potential success. The two agreed that past behaviors could be a definite barrier in present encounters with others. James made a verbal commitment to lessen the frequency of such negative behaviors. The two agreed that individual counseling provided a safe environment in which James could role play and get feedback on some new communication techniques. The psychologist got James to agree that if he succeeded as expected, he might later participate in some group social skills activities. Finally, the two agreed that by the end of the academic semester, James would be experiencing at least one positive peer interaction every day. A positive interaction was defined as one that James enjoyed and the other party did not terminate out of anger or unease.

Whatever approach is taken in analysis (and most options do involve some form of decision making or problem solving), the professional's goal during this stage is to finalize the components of an intervention plan. That plan should be one that both parties agree to and enter into voluntarily.

Intervention

Options for intervention are as varied as the clients, practitioners, and schools that become involved in individual counseling. Individual interventions often reflect the priorities of the local school administration. As noted in the first chapter, school practitioners are well aware of the number of children at risk for psychological and physical abuse. Problems voiced by students can include at-risk issues including suicide, eating disorders, physical and sexual abuse, and violence. More commonly, school practitioners hear students voice concerns about problems with teachers, classmates, and parents. Practitioners can provide individual attention and counseling that can help students address a wide variety of day-to-day and crisis situations.

Interventions similarly can vary from what might be labeled as counseling (individual sessions focusing on affective issues, for example) to activities that are guidance oriented. The professional can evaluate the extent to which client needs would benefit more from the intensity of individual counseling or the attention that can be provided in an alternative intervention, such as working with the parents to provide support to the student (see Box 4.5).

In our example, the school psychologist had a very good idea early on about what to do with James's presenting problem. Problems with peers are reported by many students, and counselors, teachers, and administrators may be able to use already developed sets of materials offered by educational publishers to help students acquire new or improved social skills. School districts and state organizations sim-

BOX 4.5. Selecting an Intervention

Verify urgency of intervention.

Review goals of counseling to insure match with overall plan of action (strategy) and components involved in implementing plan (tactics).

Select a time line that allows for implementation and takes into account student's and practitioner's schedule.

Validate selection of individual counseling as the strategy of choice.

Solicit feedback from colleague on options considered or selected.

Give student options to consider as well as your thoughts about benefits and limitations.

Reaffirm student's commitment to the change process.

Have student begin with a manageable first step.

---

ilarly provide materials dealing with social skills and peer relations. In Ms. Irons's case, a set of handouts and learning activities that she had developed over the years with students was used during her encounters with James. The psychologist, using a process developed previously of writing down a contract of what both parties were promising to do during counseling, agreed with James on the goals for counseling, the time frame within which they would work on these goals, and their commitments for the intervention phase. As described above, the intervention with James did involve him taking greater and greater responsibility for initiating positive encounters with peers. The professional was available to help James decide on daily situations within which he would like to try these new skills and experience success. James elected to work initially on his behavior in the cafeteria during lunch. Past problems in the lunchroom were a clear signal to James that he needed to make some changes to experience successful interactions.

The two planned out and then rehearsed steps for what James would do to initiate peer encounters and how he would respond to peer comments and actions. The psychologist suggested that James choose a classmate who was a good acquaintance and had James describe how in the past he would have interacted with that student during lunchroom time. After doing so, the two began to map out the components of a successful encounter. Opening comments used by James with the acquaintance were considered, potential topics to address with the peer were listed, the actual content of what could be said with the peer was reviewed, then the two sat down to role play what could have occurred.

Ms. Irons directed James's attention during the intervention by giving him homework assignments within which he would be responsible for keeping track of what he did to initiate any particular plan. Once the plan was accomplished, James would jot down a description of the event as well as his feelings both during and after what occurred.

As time progressed during the semester, the psychologist and client tried out a number of encounters. James began to initiate contact with male and female classmates in the lunchroom, the classroom, and outside of the school building. Events did not always go as he had hoped, but James maintained the energy to work through some of his difficulties. The standards by which he evaluated his success had already been defined during the analysis stage and were contained within the plan and eventual contract.

Ms. Irons remained very open to making adjustments to the intervention plan. Given the circumstances of James's problem, such flexibility was necessary to accommodate both the range of his problems and the changing nature of his skills and success in reaching out to classmates.

Any intervention program must contain similar flexibility so that both parties have the option of making adjustments, cycling back to an earlier stage of counseling, or exiting completely from the counseling option. Such flexibility gives both parties a greater sense of control of events as well as a vehicle to test out the other party to see if his/her commitment is as intense as his/her own. If the intervention plan does not seem to be working or the student is obviously not committing full energy to the effort, the practitioner can raise the question of what should be done to get the intervention plan back on track. Ultimate responsibility for implementing the plan rests with the student. By recognizing this, the professional can help the client focus attention on new behaviors to be implemented and the consequences of following through on a plan of action.

Evaluation

When the client has been working on an intervention, the practitioner will make some important decisions about whether to continue or terminate involvement. An important element of the evaluation process involves consideration of what has already occurred in the intervention. Counseling that started with defined goals and a clear set of expectations provides a context within which the practitioner and client can look back on progress that has occurred. If the counseling effort has proceeded without defining goals and objectives, the evaluation component becomes more difficult.

Knowing that success has occurred can boil down to comments

from the client, other teachers, and parents on changes in behavior or verbalizations. Often, though, changes involve much more subtle adjustments of student actions and words. One reality of working in school settings is that control of the student and monitoring of his/her actions is at best time limited. The student, after all, goes home from school every day. The professional counsels the student for a very narrow slice of the academic day. Relying on student and adult reports, the professional may not feel very confident that changes being considered are being accurately evaluated.

Recognizing such uncertainty, many practitioners have begun to emphasize documentation of student change (Box 4.6). Behavioral approaches especially have adopted strategies that have the student engage in self-monitoring or have a classroom teacher or peer keep track of specific behaviors. Change can be documented additionally in a more guidance-oriented approach that has the student engaging in a set number of job interviews, participation in a specific form of training, or sending off an agreed number of letters to college programs. The evaluation effort can document what has occurred during the intervention, the behaviors that the student has exhibited as a consequence of counseling, and the consequences of those behaviors.

Whatever approach is taken, the goal is to have some form of visible

---

BOX 4.6. Monitoring Student Progress: Points to Consider

1. Is the student satisfied with the plan? If yes, proceed. If not, consider adjustments.

2. Has the student been given adequate instructions for each element of the intervention plan? If so, does the student have written instructions or guidelines if memory fails on details?

3. Do *you* have a clear image of every action and the sequence of actions to be taken by the student? If so, is the intervention strategy described in your notes or records, listing what the student will do, when he/she will begin and complete actions, and how process and outcomes will be documented? If not, refine tactics to guarantee that actions get implemented.

4. Do you expect the student to maintain a log or other form of written verification of actions? If so, have you discussed how often you would like to touch base on progress? If no written record is to be kept by the student, are you planning to maintain documentation? If so, format of record keeping should be considered before the intervention (see Box 4.7). Regardless of your decisions on these matters, you will need to plan the next contact with the student.

5. Have you and the student agreed on what constitutes progress or success in your intervention? Does the student appear motivated to persist short of dramatic changes, or does the student need ongoing attention to foster commitment? Successful outcomes require close attention to the student's actions and motivation.

---

evidence that the plan for change occurred in a given fashion. The psychologist in our example wanted to be very certain that James not only interacted with peers as he promised but was able to increase his repertoire of effective communication skills. The option selected by the two was essentially self-monitoring and reporting of information to the staff member. Alternatives might have been to have adults in the relevant setting keep track of what James was doing in terms of approaching friends and acquaintances. Teachers in the school could have been asked to monitor James's attempts at using improved communication skills, especially if the psychologist had no opportunity to observe him in action. Trust within the counseling relationship might have reached a point at which Ms. Irons preferred to base her interpretations of James's progress solely on his reports of peer interactions.

One decision that occurs during evaluation is the choice of beginning work on a new identified problem or terminating the client–counselor relationship. Termination is a stage seldom addressed extensively in the counseling literature but a very important one, especially with students. When confidence and motivation have been increased by working with an adult, the student is understandably reluctant to leave the nest and be more independent. The trade-off for the professional is building confidence and competency without increasing the dependency of the client. No fixed guidelines exist for how to walk this line effectively all the time, but school practitioners do report a variety of strategies by which they are successful. The essence of the strategies boils down to the practitioner reinforcing the notion that the client maintains final responsibility for actions and decisions that follow the counseling activities. Problem ownership is defined from the start, and a portion of the client's sense of competency comes from always having the option of pushing on with an intervention or waiting for alternative courses of action.

Evaluation of success is a desirable goal, but evaluation of efforts that failed can be similarly instructive. Both parties can begin to understand how they individually and collectively contributed to some of the limitations of the intervention (Box 4.7). Reflecting on those limitations and understanding what occurred may be the motivation for the student to attempt a new course of action. The professional can learn a number of lessons from failure to help the student. He/she may have confronted some very real limits of expertise and choose in the future to refer students with similar problems to other professionals. The staff member may be motivated similarly to seek out training and experiences that will enhance expertise.

BOX 4.7. Items for a Counseling Evaluation Form

Record of contact (process of counseling)
  Documentation of each planned activity
  a. Activity 1
  b. Activity 2, etc.

  Documentation of target and completion dates of activities
  a. Target date to initiate activity 1
  b. Actual date initiated activity 1 (on time or late?)
  c. Promised completion date of activity 1
  d. Actual completion date of activity 1, etc.

  Confirmation (if agrees) of documentation items
  a. Indication of who can confirm documentation items above
  b. Otherwise, sign-off of student or counselor

Outcomes
  Planned changes
  a. Describe outcomes to be accomplished.
  b. Assess degree of accomplishment of outcomes.
  c. Note actions if plan was simply attendance at function.

  Unplanned changes in behavior, affect, thinking (for example, self-esteem)
  a. Describe and assess unanticipated positive outcomes.
  b. Describe and assess unanticipated negative consequences.

USEFUL TECHNIQUES FOR INDIVIDUAL COUNSELING

A number of techniques and strategies have proven useful to school practitioners who have engaged in counseling interventions. Within this section, information on behavioral and Adlerian techniques that have been influential in current counseling practices are discussed.

Behavioral Techniques

The behavioral approach to counseling has had its adherents and critics. Although behavioral approaches have proven very effective with students in a variety of situations, some observers have been hesitant to adopt techniques and strategies because of the perception that behavioral approaches are too manipulative or simplistic in affecting student behaviors. Rather than engaging in a discussion of the merits of either side of this argument, the authors will review a few of the components of the behavioral approach to counseling that can be effective during individual counseling, regardless of the counseling philosophy of the professional (Box 4.8).

BOX 4.8. Behavioral Applications in Individual Counseling

Establishing a baseline

Specificity in behavioral description, goal setting, and evaluation

Contracting for behavioral change

Using reinforcement procedures to strengthen behaviors

Using extinction/ignoring to weaken behaviors

Training students to monitor their own change programs

An important notion in the behavioral approach is that of establishing a baseline. By baseline, the professional would be defining exactly how the student was behaving, thinking, or feeling at a given time prior to the counseling involvement. Gathering baseline data involves the student, classroom teacher, counselor, or others in documenting what the student is doing and saying. How the documentation occurs, of course, is influenced by the presenting problem, available time to establish baseline information, and preferences of the professional. Baseline can be as simple as having students report how many times they think about running away from home or documenting the number of times that they hit a sibling or the number of times that they blurt out a comment in jest during a classroom activity. The intent of baseline is to establish behavior in terms of frequency or other relevant dimensions (latency, duration, etc.). By having a baseline, both parties are able to document progress that the student makes over the course of an intervention.

Another behavioral notion of interest to all counselors is specificity. Baseline data gathering allows school practitioners to pin down behaviors and cognitions to the most concrete level. Being specific, however, is at the heart of all behavioral strategies. Problem definition, the establishment of the goals and objectives by the adult and student, includes agreement on just what is occurring and how independent observers could agree on the behavior actually occurring.

In an example from an elementary school, a classroom teacher was talking to the school nurse about a particular child, Jonathan, in her class. Jonathan's problem, according to the teacher, was excessive shyness. As the nurse listened to the teacher, he was unclear about just what was being defined as shyness. After talking for a few minutes, the teacher specified that shyness for her meant not talking to classmates in group settings, only in one-on-one encounters. The nurse commented that other children had similar hesitations in speaking out at group settings and tried to find out if the student's behavior was interfering with any academic goals.

For this teacher, group participation was critical, as most learning activities were structured within groups. Very few options were available for individual learning. The teacher decided to chat with the child and to see if Jonathan had a similar perception of shyness within group but not individual settings. Thus, in this situation, what was considered a problem evolved from a quite vague label of shyness to a more specific one of frequency of conversation with peers in a group setting.

Specificity and concreteness in describing behaviors assist the professional throughout the duration of counseling, letting changes as they occur be easy to document and thus to evaluate. An additional notion promoted by many behaviorists is that of contracts. Contracts are a straightforward way in which both parties can define the dimensions of the change process. The professional can list what he/she will be doing to work with the student, the student can list what he/she has set as a goal and promises to do to achieve that goal, and both can define how they will deal with success or failure of the plan. Contracts can be formal (written) or informal (oral), serving the purpose of clarifying (being specific) what each can expect of the other in the time frame within which they will be working together. Contracts also serve the purpose of alerting other parties, such as other teachers and parents, to the concerns being addressed during counseling. By serving as a record of agreement and accomplishments, the contract will help remind both parties of what has been promised and planned and how events are progressing. The practitioner and client can always change components or time frames referenced in the contract.

A note should be made at this point of the idea of reinforcement that is central to behavioral approaches. Reinforcement (and the related notion of reward) is a term that triggers resistance in some observers. The idea behind reinforcement is to recognize that under certain conditions, the child can be guided toward change by providing contingencies specific to the student's behavior. For example, in a very simple fashion, a plan might be for the student to stay in his/her seat during the classroom period and, in recognition of that behavior, be provided with 10 minutes of free time during a subsequent class period. What arouses the attention of some observers is the perception that the student is being rewarded for behavior that should be occurring anyway. Behaviorists would not necessarily argue with that perception but would recognize that if the child's behavior has been a problem, then circumstances in that child's environment must be manipulated to achieve desired goals. If students can be manipulated to behave in ways we perceive as more positive, then providing them with access to free time can be seen as the price we pay to achieve our goals. Again, our intent is not to criticize or applaud any specific approach to counseling but simply to argue that some of the techniques being described have proven quite effective in changing student behavior.

A final technique that has proven successful is that of self-monitoring, mentioned above in James's intervention. Training students to monitor themselves has proven to be a viable alternative to monitoring students' behaviors ourselves. Although all students can't be expected to monitor their own actions adequately, most students do have an awareness of themselves and a commitment to working with the professional and can be trained effectively to keep track of thoughts, actions, or emotions that they are experiencing. Self-monitoring techniques have been evaluated by a number of investigators and have been found to be sound alternatives to documentation provided by outside observers.

An additional example of training a student to monitor himself/herself comes from an individual counseling program developed by a middle school teacher. The professional, Ms. Borowski, was working with a student, Ronald, who had a great deal of difficulty finishing assignments and staying in his seat. Ronald had a number of other problems involving family and peer relations, but one important component of his work with Ms. Borowski was centered on his attention during class. Part of the work with Ronald in the classroom involved training him to monitor his actions, especially staying seated and completing assignments. Ronald was taught to keep a simple checklist in one corner of his desk on which he kept track of each small component of his assignment. Ms. Borowski provided assignments to Ronald that were broken into clearly identified sections, allowing Ronald to maintain a check on his progress during each class session. Ronald needed such assistance because one of his problems that cut across several classroom settings was organization and time management. Training him to monitor his actions and take responsibility for reporting his progress to the teacher was an important form of preparation that he eventually did generalize to additional classroom settings. Self-monitoring can involve checking off accomplishments as in Ronald's case or recording such information using any system of documentation for a teacher, staff member, or administrator.

Many other behavioral techniques have been integrated into the counseling process. One good source that provides an in-depth look at a behavioral approach to counseling is that of Bergan (1979), whose text also reviews the behavioral consultation approach.

Adlerian Approaches

Alfred Adler's influence on counseling has been profound and has extended to all aspects of school practice. Adler's ideas on discipline and misbehavior have served as the basis for approaches to parent education, discipline planning, and teacher preparation. A few of his ideas that are especially useful during counseling are reviewed below (Box 4.9).

Adler emphasized the distinction between encouragement and praise. His distinction is relevant to counseling because our work with students needs to take account of process as well as product. Encouragement is seen as what we would say to students to keep them working, keep them on task, and keep them motivated. Praise is an activity that we use to reflect on the accomplishments or products of that child's endeavor. Students experiencing problems, however, often are deficient in terms of product and need to be motivated or directed around process issues. Encouragement that focuses on how a student works rather than what he/she accomplishes can thus prove to be important during counseling. Many of the effective communication skills discussed in Chapter 3 reinforce the idea that we must center our attention whenever possible on what the student is doing at any given time rather than delaying our reinforcement until he/she has accomplished our intervention goals. Encouragement is a useful concept, one that we can extend beyond the counseling situation to our discussions with parents and colleagues to encourage them to recognize the process of a student's work.

A second idea that has proven relevant to counseling is that of logical consequences. Adler and his followers such as Dinkmeyer and Dreikurs have written extensively on the distinction between logical consequences and punishment. Punishment involves the application of a consequence to students but in a way that may not be directly related to what they have done. Logical consequences, by definition, will be our response to students in such a way that it is clear to them that they know that we are reacting to their particular behavior and

---

BOX 4.9. Adlerian Applications in Individual Counseling

Emphasis on encouragement rather than praise

Training students to recognize the distinction between logical consequences (and natural consequences) and punishment

Promoting democratic structures in the home and the classroom

Emphasizing personal responsibility and problem ownership

Dealing with the sources of a student's problem as well as the problem itself

---

our response is intended to signal what they could do differently. For example, if a child is throwing a pencil around the room, punishment might involve placing the student in a corner of the room or writing 10 times on the blackboard that he/she will never throw pencils again. Writing your name on the blackboard or standing in the corner are events not directly related to pencil throwing and are instead a reflection of our frustration with the child. On the other hand, if we work with that student after taking the pencil away to have him/her think about the problem behavior and to make a commitment to behave differently in the future, our discipline will be a logical response to the behavior of concern.

Establishing logical consequences may be easier to describe than to achieve, as we have experienced. The school practitioner working with the child has to be quite creative to think through any given difficulty that the student is presenting and come up with a consequence that logically ties into the student's actions. Understanding and applying logical consequences can be a goal in working with the other important people in the child's life (such as parents) to help them to structure their interactions to guide the student toward new behaviors and to maintain motivation to behave appropriately.

Related to encouragement and logical consequences is Adler's idea of the family or classroom as a democracy. Adler stresses that within a democratic structure, all participants are more likely to feel a sense of participation and commitment than in alternative structures such as autocratic or authoritarian classrooms. Helping a student plan for the future can occur whether or not the student works within a democratic structure. However, one conflict that arises in trying to help a student occurs when the adults in that student's life argue that everyone is equal and all should work together and yet dramatically restrict thoughts and actions of that student. When the student does not perceive having a choice in behavior, one common outcome is what Adler calls misbehavior.

Getting the student to promise change can be enhanced, Adlerians argue, when democratic structures exist for that child. Such structures do not exist automatically and must be nurtured by the practitioner when appropriate. Programs for teacher training and parent education exist that focus on the Adlerian notions of democratic structures and how to help students experience encouragement as well as logical consequences. Materials by Dinkmeyer and Dreikurs noted in Appendix B are good examples of the Adlerian option.

All the notions discussed above under the Adlerian section reduce to the idea of personal responsibility, or what some people call problem ownership. Adler was very aware of the difficulty that some students have in growing up. Often adults in a student's life try to protect him/her or to shield him/her from taking responsibility in everyday life. Adler's notion was to not expect responsibility until we let students have the opportunity to exhibit it. Adults, thus, must take the lead in being sure that the student has many opportunities to recognize his/her abilities and to behave in a way that gains attention for being responsible.

The idea of problem ownership is closely related to responsibility. When difficulty does occur, say between a child and an adult, the idea of problem ownership is to establish who has primary responsibility for initiating problem resolution. If the student is having difficulty with the classroom teacher, problem ownership would involve both parties recognizing that something is going on that involves both participants in a coordinated way. Problem ownership is established when both parties review what has occurred and can determine who maintains the initiative for dealing with the difficulty. If the student is seen by the teacher as owning the problem but the student does not want to address an issue, the teacher must make the decision of how he/she will act.

Readers are encouraged to consult either Adler's writings, which are addressed primarily at nonschool issues, or the writings of his followers such as Dinkmeyer and Dreikurs, who focus their attention on the agendas of public education (see Appendix A). As argued above, Adlerian ideas have had a pervasive influence on parent education, school services, and counseling. Knowledge of Adler's ideas will assist the professional in understanding clients and establishing an agenda for service.

COMMON STRATEGIES FOR DEALING WITH STUDENT PROBLEMS

An important distinction to consider at this point is that between crisis interventions and proactive interventions. Definitions for crisis intervention vary widely, depending on the writer. Crisis interventions are intended to address immediate and pressing concerns in such a way that action occurs quickly. Proactive interventions, by definition, are preventive in nature, preparing the student for potential difficulties dealing with school or home environments.

When remediation is the priority, individual counseling offers the option of expediently gathering information on problems of concern, focusing the attention of the client on what can be done, and starting a course of action that can help resolve difficulties. Proactive or preventive strategies are less likely to occur in an individual than in a group setting within which preparing participants for possible difficulties appears feasible. We do not rule out the possibility of a preventive agenda being established for an individual counseling session but do recognize that remedial strategies and agendas will apply to the vast majority of situations.

What follows is a brief review of some of the agenda items addressed in individual counseling. The priorities for such service do not exclude serving the student in other ways, such as through group counseling or nonschool types of programming.

Social skills and the problems that evolve from difficulties in communication and behavior are an important agenda item for young as well as older students. Whether the student is shy or aggressive, the practitioner can deal with the difficulties being experienced using the individual option. Increasingly, schools have available social skills training programs, but at this point such programs often are restricted to children within special education programs. On the other hand, all students at some point get into difficulty in relating to others, both adults and peers. When such relationship problems interfere with other priorities of the school, such as academics, individual counseling can be directed to helping the student establish better control over behaviors. The child who talks out too much, the child who is too aggressive with friends as well as other classmates, the child who just doesn't seem to want to get involved in any activities can be assisted through the individual counseling option.

A second group of students that come to our attention is that of students with school attendance and related problems. Students even at the lowest grade levels develop patterns of truancy that can result in work with the entire family. School attendance is a concern to administrators and teachers, who develop their programs based on full attendance. As students approach the juvenile years, truancy and other behaviors such as running away from home bring them to the attention of juvenile authorities. Events in the adolescent years bring with them complications of working with parents who may be uninterested in working with their child. Individual counseling provides a context within which some trust can be established with the client so that problem solving to keep the student in school or at home can be negotiated. Individual counseling can offer an environment within which the student feels safe to talk about problems.

Truancy, running away, and problems at home are not easy to resolve. Individual counseling can at best work with a small number of students, those who are willing to give the schools a chance to help them resolve some of their own ideas about what is best for them.

Students, especially in adolescence, can get into increasingly negative interactions with peers and adults, bringing them to the attention of school and community authorities. Students who engage in vandalism and forms of law breaking in the community are only some of the students at risk of future difficulty. Other students might behave in ways that place them at danger of their lives. Drug and alcohol abuse, driving at high speeds, and other forms of life-threatening activities all are common among some sets of students. Problems with parents become more difficult for the adolescent to resolve as the issue of independence becomes central to their plans for the future.

Schools are cautious about intervening in many of these situations, especially on an individual counseling level. We know very little about the potential efficacy of individual counseling for any of these concerns. However, until we know more about school and nonschool group programs and their success in dealing with these issues, the individual counseling option should be pursued. The counselor has only to talk to case officers assigned to juvenile justice programs to realize the limitations of most approaches that have been tried in response to vandalism, property destruction, drug and alcohol abuse, etc. The behaviors that lead to these difficulties in adolescents have roots in the family during the child's earliest years. Preventive programs offer the opportunity to address some of the behaviors and thoughts that reinforce negative behaviors.

The individual counseling approach does provide an important dimension of response to such problem areas. Practitioners who have the alternative of individual work with a student have an important form of leverage with clients. Focused individual attention provided in a way that elicits trust and caring is a very profound form of service. Intensity of feelings and reactions can deepen during that exchange. When the student is open to the influence of those interactions, individual counseling can work very quickly to deal with difficulties and prepare students to deal better with their own world.

CONCLUSIONS

The individual approach to counseling students offers many advantages to the practitioner. Time with the client can be concentrated on the presenting issues, services can move quickly without the distractions of other children being present, and the adult can implement strategies appropriate only to the one-on-one context. Limits on individual counseling relate to available time and energy of the student and professional, service priorities of the individual school, and parental support for such services.

Training is necessary before the school practitioner can, with confidence and skill, approach the demands of individual counseling. Preservice and in-service experiences may have prepared the professional for the strategies involved in the individual approach, or such training can be sought so that services can be effectively provided.

Services to the individual student thus become part of the general structure of services to the entire student body. Such services can be coordinated with others being delivered to the students. Keeping administrators, colleagues, and parents informed of the content of services can be the professional's responsibility as part of a plan for services being attempted with the student.

The professional growth of the practitioner will be influenced by actions taken with the client. As new strategies for enhancing change are implemented, the educator will better understand the limits of his/her effectiveness. Getting to know children within the intensity of individual counseling is a growth experience for both parties. Because of the benefits for both parties, the individual counseling option should be supported as a form of intervention in all schools.

5

Group Counseling

Group counseling is an activity that usually is conducted by trained professionals within an educational setting. This chapter provides a condensed description of the goals of group counseling suggested by certain theories, a review of the usefulness of group counseling with certain students, and finally a series of practical suggestions for educators who wish to accomplish specific goals through a series of meetings with a group of students.

There may very well be certain conditions under which a teacher, school psychologist, or social worker will decide to conduct group counseling. The suggested readings (see Appendix B) provide detailed descriptions for educators who desire additional material. One important consideration, just as with individual counseling, is to identify a trusted colleague who can be counted on to support you, to listen to concerns, and to give you feedback as the counseling group progresses. It is necessary that an educator enlist the support of a trusted colleague to serve as a consultant before a new group gets under way and during the life of the group.

The objectives for any group significantly determine how the leader will function, the main activities of the group, and expected behaviors by successful members of the group. As an example, discussion groups as used by many teachers often have as a purpose the goal of increasing student awareness of opinions held by classmates on a designated topic. The leader functions to draw in as many opinions as possible, to allow students to complete their ideas without interruption, and to provide summaries where appropriate. Successful members of discussion groups express their opinions, listen to other members, and cooperate in order to maximize the discussion within the group.

Just as in a discussion group, the purposes of a counseling group will influence expectations for the leader and for members. Recently, writers on group counseling have zeroed in on quite specific purposes for different groups. Support groups for children undergoing the experience of parents getting a divorce, for students who need to develop social skills or study skills, or for students transferring into a new school are some examples of groups with a specific purpose.

The need for group counseling is great since students look to peers for acceptance and for support. Unfortunately, recent surveys have indicated a serious lack of groups being provided in many educational settings (Ehly, Dustin, & Forsyth, 1985). School psychologists, teachers, and administrators may wish to help a group of students accomplish selected goals as indicated above.

Before deciding that group counseling is the service of choice, the educator should consult with a trusted professional and obtain a commitment from this colleague to be available for advice and further consultation as the group develops. Advanced preparation can allow the professional to begin the planning necessary for a successful counseling group. Box 5.1 lists some of the considerations of the physical environment of the group, just one factor to be considered before a group meets. One important area in which planning is important concerns the outcomes of a counseling group, that is, just what is supposed to happen?

GOALS OF GROUP COUNSELING

Certain theories from counseling and psychotherapy have been widely applied to groups. Several texts offer thorough descriptions of all

---

BOX 5.1. Desirable Physical Arrangements for a Group

1. Is there privacy for members? If a member gets upset and leaves the group, or if a student comes late, how noticeable will this be to other students?
2. Is the setting pleasant? Even if limited by institutional priorities for paint or by monochromatic drabness, can the leader put up posters or provide some splash of color?
3. Are seating arrangements comfortable? Have arrangements been made for the access of each group member to the space?
4. Is there enough silence so that members can hear each other? Are ringing phones, banging pipes, and movement of students and staff of such nature that members will have difficulty concentrating?
5. Groups with purposes that are likely to require note taking—study skills groups or problem-solving groups—will need desks or space for students to write.

---

the major theories (Corey, 1981; George & Dustin, 1988) that have influenced group counseling. Three major theories—Rogerian, Adlerian, and behavioral—are briefly examined here with a focus on goals and objectives. These theories are considered for their relevance to group counseling.

Rogerian Groups

Rogerian counseling has frequently been applied within group settings (Rogers, 1972). The goals of such groups emphasize intrapersonal awareness and insights into members' feelings and self-perceptions. Members slowly come to trust each other and the leader and learn to examine their own doubts and capabilities while in the group. Closeness among members leads to increased self-disclosure and risk taking as members share increasingly more information about themselves. The insights that result help the group accomplish such goals as increased self-understanding, self-acceptance, and self-regard. Such insights are the expected outcomes for Rogerian counseling. Box 5.2 lists how a Rogerian leader might help the group set goals.

BOX 5.2. How a Rogerian Leader Might Set Goals

In an educational setting in the 1990s, no doubt a practitioner will need to be able to describe the purposes of a group in sufficient detail for administrators, teachers, and perhaps parents to understand. Therefore, the notion of an ambiguous situation that is viewed as a starting place for some encounter groups, where students are confused about why they have been sent for and just what is supposed to happen, is unlikely. However, a Rogerian leader would strongly believe that students will value a group more if they have been able to have a voice in rules and norms for the group.

Leader statements might include the following:

"So. Do you other students also believe that I should be the one to decide what we are supposed to do?"

"I'd like to hear what some of you students think about a group where students could set the rules."

"Jerry believes that we would be a good group if we had no rules. What do some of you others think?"

"It sounds like, Terry, that if you don't know what members are supposed to do in a group, then you don't know what you're supposed to talk about. Is that right?"

"So far today it seems we have had confusion about this group. I hoped you would help set the rules, and several of you aren't sure. Would you think about our problem until next time?"

Students in a Rogerian counseling group learn that their leader will accept their feelings and other personal disclosures. As each member observes the acceptance given to all members, he/she finds it easier to open up in the group. Insight into the member's own feelings and self-view follow.

For example, at first, Lindy was apprehensive about her new group. What had she gotten herself into? What did the leader mean when he told her that the group would allow her to learn more about herself? Now it was the first meeting. When she first spoke, Lindy wasn't sure what she had said. But now she heard herself say, "I think this is going well. I appreciate hearing each of you tell about yourselves. I have been having trouble in school, and I think I need a place to think and to clarify my goals. I hope this group will be the place. I can tell you for sure that I'll be here next week at the next meeting."

As other members hear individuals such as Lindy gradually express their comfort with the group, they too begin to open up and to share in the group's activities. Insights into one's own behavior follow this sharing and the increase in self-exploration by the group's members.

Adlerian Groups

Adlerian theorists have described meeting-by-meeting goals and activities for parents and students engaged in group counseling (Dinkmeyer, Pew, & Dinkmeyer, 1979). The reader might be interested in examining these Adlerian-influenced materials for an idea of the complex planning and specificity of goals that have been developed for group counseling. See Appendix B for major sources of information on Adlerian theory and applications.

Goals for Adlerian counseling include insight, as did Rogerian counseling, but the desired insights are expanded beyond the affect area of Rogerian groups to include increased self-understanding about the members' thinking and behavior. Adlerians assume that each of us has a "life script" that was developed early in life. This script includes basic life goals that individuals develop in response to their family situation and their perceived role in the family. By school age, the script is developed but usually outside one's awareness. Therefore, a group can help increase understanding as members explore their own goals and come to understand possible motives for their behavior. Box 5.3 lists some of the elements of a life script.

An example may help clarify how goals can gradually be understood and then changed. Monique is a fourth grade student who constantly is at the teacher's side. If she doesn't have questions, she

BOX 5.3. Elements of a Life Script

By the age of 5 or 6, Adlerians believe, individuals are well on their way to patterned responses to life's challenges. Individuals start responding to not getting their way early in life. The student who withdraws when frustrated, the one who gets blustery and insists on immediate results, will tend to repeat this style over and over.

Individuals seem to persist with:

1. A certain activity level: amount of overt movement in a certain period of time; amount of sleep needed; attention span
2. Length of time they will try or will persist in frustrating activity
3. Tendency to seek out others to help them
4. Amount of time spent analyzing or thinking about problem
5. Tendency for direct action
6. Whether they see authority as a source of support, a solution, or with distrust
7. Amount of confidence that they will successfully solve a problem

---

has something to show the teacher. Exasperated, the teacher began to have Monique meet with a few other third and fourth grade students in the hopes that other students could provide alternative behaviors for Monique.

Monique exhibited the same behavior in the group. One day, rather than react as she did in class, the teacher stopped giving directions and addressed Monique.

"Monique, I think you want my attention."

Startled, Monique looked at the teacher and then looked away.

Before anyone could say anything else, another group member stated, "That's nothing new. That's what she does all day long."

The teacher responded, "What about it, Monique? Do you recognize that you do this quite often?"

Quietly, Monique responded, "Yes."

"Well, that is one thing I want you to work on in this group. The other children are going to help you. Perhaps you can learn other ways to get my attention without interrupting me and the other children. Do you think we can do that?"

Goals that are quite relevant for students include the need for attention, the need for revenge, the desire for power, and a need to show helplessness (Corsini, 1984). These goals are rarely within the student's awareness, and a rather long-range group program with consistent yet kindly reminders can result in behavior change, which is another desired goal for Adlerian groups.

Behavioral Groups

Behavioral groups have specific goals that are publicly negotiated in the group by each member. Often, the group leader is very task centered and keeps the group focused on the specific learning contracts of each member. The overall purpose of most behavioral groups is to use the group climate to promote individual behavior change. The behavioral group leader provides praise and promotes mutual support by group members for the gradual improvement experienced by each member.

Jerry, for example, in his eighth grade support group, which has a behavioral orientation, has set the goal of getting to school on time. The leader now helps the group explore how Jerry can accomplish this.

As one or two members volunteer to become involved, the group begins to offer the active support and reinforcement for successful changes that characterize an effective behavioral counseling group. For example, Jess says that he used to be "late all the time" too. Jerry asks Jess what happened to get him to school on time. Gradually Jerry seems to open up to suggestions much more than he had when the leader made suggestions. Such improvement as happened with Jerry is often compared with behavior at the start of the group. Box 5.4 describes the use of a baseline in a group.

BOX 5.4. Behavioral Change in Group Counseling

As soon as individual members seem to understand the ground rules for group membership, the leader can begin to identify specific change strategies with a single member. As the group sees progress—that is, when the first member agrees that he/she wants to start changing a specific behavior—then the group will suddenly hold more interest and attractiveness for the members.

To begin the process, the leader could start with a member who is known to be highly motivated to change a behavior.

"Tell us a little bit about what behavior is needing change, Dickie."

As the leader helps Dickie get specific about what type of behavior frequency would be more desirable, the first assignment is made.

"Here is a card, Dickie. Can the rest of you see it? I want you to check each time it happens Monday. The first column is Monday, then how often Tuesday, and we'll be together again next Wednesday. Do you understand?"

At the next meeting the leader must follow through and check with Dickie about the frequency of the behavior. Optimally, a goal is set then, and Dickie is directed to continue to count. The same card becomes a record of how well the member is doing and, hence, of how well the group has been helpful.

Implementing Goals in Groups

We now turn to a description of just how goals can be implemented with specific students. What is the expected impact of a group on its members?

Effective group counseling will have an impact on each individual member in the areas of attitude and behavior change. Increased self-understanding for a student can occur through the feedback and advice of other group members, even in those cases where admonishments and lectures from helping adults seem to have failed. Because the group member is placed among peers, group counseling can open up an individual to the same statements that were previously rejected. Although students are influenced by adults, by school age the peer group is especially influential. It makes sense to utilize this influence in peer groups.

An effective group counselor can train members of the group to give specific feedback in a manner that can be understood and acted on. When members help the individual identify a specific area of behavior that causes problems for the individual and for the other students, the problem seems real. What may have been seen by the student as only something bothering a teacher now becomes the student's problem as group members indicate how much they also dislike the behavior.

TEACHER: It sounds as if you are telling Jerry that you don't like it when he runs around the room during reading.
MEMBER 1: Right, he bothers us and sometimes grabs my pencil.
OTHERS: Yeah. That's right.
TEACHER: Jerry, does this reaction from the others surprise you?

In a group climate in which acceptance of each member has been developed, members can explore their own reactions to each other and, even more important, explore what they think about how their actions are affecting others.

TEACHER: Jerry, it sounds as though the students don't like your running around when they are working. What do you have to say to them?
JERRY: I don't know. I don't always bother you other guys.
MEMBER 2: Just your running around bothers us.

Finally, those groups focusing on behavior change offer an even greater opportunity for the impact of the group to make itself felt on individuals. Box 5.5 offers a checklist for a school practitioner to consider as the decision is made whether to offer group counseling to a student. As stated previously, the goals of any counseling group strongly affect the activities of the group. In those cases in which individual behavior change is a goal for the group, then the counseling can take on a special focus as individuals decide to try to change because some of the group members want them to.

Sometimes educators may use a collection of students as a convenience. Not all gatherings of students, even those in which the adult in charge desires changes in student behavior, are counseling. For example, the reader may be familiar with a situation in which several students are kept together after school. Occasionally, the proctor or "leader" may charge the students in a manner such as the following: "Now I don't want any of you to repeat that behavior [which resulted in the detention]. I don't want to see any of you in here after school again."

Such admonitions, even if accompanied by threats, are not the best method to accomplish behavior change, even in group counseling. The time and careful planning required for group counseling would not be worthwhile if threats worked.

In addition to having a group of interested members, there are other characteristics that can help the facilitator ensure success. Students who ask to be in a group are, of course, the ideal. Even when other staff members have referred students, the group leader can obtain commitment from students to be in the group after explaining

---

BOX 5.5. Checklist for Group Membership

When trying to determine whether a student might benefit from membership in a group, consider:

1. Whether an appropriate group exists. If yes, is it an open group, one that accepts members as it goes? Will the members likely be of help to the student under consideration?
2. Whether the needs of the student would be likely to benefit from suggestions and support from other students.
3. What was the reaction of the student when the subject of group membership was broached? Counseling is designed to be voluntary. Instances where students are coerced into counseling are unlikely to prove successful.
4. Does the student seem willing to follow the rules for membership, or whatever guidelines are being used with the group? Obtaining commitment before allowing the student to attend the first group seems important.
5. Is the student willing to attend one group meeting to try it out?
6. Have the necessary permissions been obtained?

---

expectations for group membership. Although there are groups in which members are forced to participate, for example, inpatient groups and substance abuse groups, such groups are difficult and are not recommended unless the leader has a great deal of experience.

Although a step-by-step description for successful group counseling is found at the end of this chapter, strategies for obtaining behavior change can now be considered.

By interviewing prospective group members prior to the beginning of the group, the facilitator can determine the interest of the prospective member and the chances of successful behavior change. Even more important, the expectations for the group can be made clear. Clarity of expectation is so important that the group leader needs to explain to each group member the goals and what is expected of each group member before the group starts and again at the first meeting.

TEACHER: In this group, Tyrone, each of the members will be working to change some of his actions. You will be expected to help the other members and also to make some changes yourself. Do you think you'd be interested in attending at least one meeting?

The facilitator needs to help the members warm up to the task and to each other. The accepting nature of the leader helps set the tone for the group and for subsequent meetings. The group is a place where a member can be honest and where members will try to help. The gradual trust and caring among group members set group counseling apart from other types of groups such as learning groups and discussion groups and form a necessary prerequisite for subsequent change.

As members begin to self-disclose and to open up in the group, many students will blame others for their troubles and for their being in the group and will deny much personal responsibility for their actions. The effective facilitator needs to accept this tendency for some to blame others and to avoid responsibility yet nudge the group away from griping so that goals for new behavior can be set.

TEACHER: It sounds as if several of you think that I am picking on you. But I notice that each of your stories has one thing in common. When you don't complete your assignment, that's when the trouble occurs. What about you, Dickie? Does this tend to happen when you don't have your homework done?"

As individual members establish personal goals for behavior change, the group can help as a monitor, a source of encouragement, and a cheering section. Gradually each member uses group time to report back his/her progress on behavior changes and to continue setting goals on the way to success.

For example, Dickie decided he would finish his arithmetic before he would allow himself to play with the other boys after school, even if that meant staying after school. At first the group was skeptical: "Oh, you won't do it." "You're only telling that to Mrs. Brown; you don't mean it."

But gradually the group became impressed and told Dickie so. "You're really doing it." "You don't get yelled at any more like you used to."

TEACHER: What about it, Dickie? Have you been able to get your arithmetic done?

DICKIE: Yeah. I have. But these guys help. Yesterday I wanted to go play kick ball, but Todd reminded me that I hadn't finished my stuff.

The member-to-member advice that occurs among students has been viewed as extremely important (Yalom, 1985). The impact of successful group counseling that can result from member-to-member advice is now briefly described.

Interpersonal learning is often a goal of teachers who may find that the regular classroom does not provide enough opportunity to try to understand the student, explore the student's view of the problem, offer alternative behaviors for the student, and follow through and guide the student's attempts to change. Promotion of interpersonal learning and skill development through such member-to-member exchanges is exactly what group counseling can do best. Individuals can help each other as they react to what others are saying and to what they have observed in the group.

Modeling has frequently been used to teach complex behaviors such as high jumping or passing a baton in track relays. In group counseling, as members develop caring for each other, modeling among members can be a powerful source of new behaviors and can encourage individuals to try alternatives. Box 5.6 shows how modeling can be used in group counseling.

For many members, the group can become a primary source of support. Students who don't receive much encouragement or don't have many settings in which they feel important become excellent group members as they experience interpersonal warmth.

Finally, effective group counseling can result in specific changes in behaviors and skills. Group counseling has been used to teach social skills, study skills, stress reduction, and other specific skill areas (Duncan & Gumaer, 1980; Lieberman, 1980). Such a group in which specific skills are being learned is quite different from many class-

BOX 5.6. Modeling in the Group

Modeling is often a helpful way for individual members to be of assistance to each other. One rather straightforward way to utilize modeling is when role play in the group becomes difficult.

"O.K., it seems that Amy is having trouble expressing herself to her older sister. Ruth, I thought you played a very good older sister. I can tell you have experience. Stay in that role. Who in the group would like to show Amy how they would talk to her sister? Roz? O.K."

"Now remember that Amy wants to stand up for herself without crying, but also without calling her sister names. Have you got it? Ruth, are you ready?"

"Amy, watch Roz to see if she does anything that you would like to do with your sister."

As members try out different aspects of role plays, certain individuals become models for behaviors desired by others. In addition, the other members become coaches and cheerleaders, encouraging the individual to "try harder—I know you can do it."

rooms since the leader/facilitator utilizes different activities and uses the other learners in a manner different from the traditional classroom. The advantage of teaching skills in group counseling is the important role given to the other learners in the group.

In summary, selected theories from counseling and psychotherapy suggest that positive change is possible for each member of a group if certain group activities occur, for example, group leader acceptance and empathy for Rogerians and clear focus on task using members to reinforce each other for behavioral leaders. The expected changes for individuals experiencing successful group counseling occur in the areas of attitude and behavioral change. In addition, members learn from and about each other through their participation.

USEFULNESS OF GROUP COUNSELING

One major justification for group counseling seems to be that the group leader spends time with a group of students rather than with one at a time. However, this apparent efficiency often does not save on the actual time the adult is involved. Because of the time spent in planning, the very real need for consultation with a colleague, and the possibility of increased requests for individual time from members of the group, the leader may not save time over what would be required in individual counseling. Counseling groups do offer an effective use of professional time for those cases in which other interventions have failed. In addition, counseling groups may provide a service that is needed by some students and that previously has not been satisfactorily provided.

For example, Mr. Judd, a shop teacher, became quite exasperated with the rudeness and lack of manners among the eighth graders in his classes. After attending a workshop about how two teachers had been successful teaching social skills in a group setting, Mr. Judd talked with a counselor in his building. He learned that there were no social skills groups underway. The counselor agreed with Mr. Judd about the need, especially among some of the eighth graders, for some social training but declared that the two counselors were just too busy and had no plans to start such a group. Somewhat tentatively, Mr. Judd selected six of the worst offenders and began a social skills group with the encouragement and help of the counselor.

The actual decision to place a particular student in a counseling group may be the result of a great deal of trial and error and even exasperation by the professional. For example, Mr. Judd was more than frustrated by three of the eighth graders whom he decided to place in his first group. Group counseling, although not magic and certainly not among the easiest of interventions, may prove to be an effective service for certain students.

Among the student characteristics that may suggest membership in groups are the following. Belligerent, aggressive students who may engage in bullying behavior are one type of student for whom group interventions may prove helpful. Such students often elicit aggressive, bullying responses from educators, such as threats and ultimatums. Often, the student has learned the aggressive, bullying behavior at home, and such responses from educators serve to reinforce for the child that such behaviors are effective.

An effective group counselor will accept the bully, even while setting firm guidelines for whatever behaviors will be tolerated in the group. Usually aggressive students will be placed in heterogeneous groups rather than in an entire group of belligerent students. However, the patience and consistency required for success will provide a challenge for any facilitator. Activities to promote social learning in which specific behavioral goals are included would seem to offer a promising area of service to such students.

Quiet, shy students may very well respond positively to group counseling. As other students come to care for them and express concern and interest in the quiet student, attitude change and subsequent behavior change may occur. Quiet students often respond very positively to the opportunity to offer suggestions and support to others and may develop a strong attachment to the group through their efforts at helping other students.

There will, of course, be many students for whom a teacher will desire behavior change. However, group counseling interventions are predicated on voluntary group membership. Research indicates that the greatest change occurs for group members who are highly motivated to attend the group. Efforts at requesting or even coercing others to change are not counseling. Instead, a teacher can consider a counseling group for students who exhibit certain behaviors and who volunteer to participate. Groups in which students are coerced to attend cannot be called counseling groups. The clarity of expectation that is helpful for successful groups can help students decide whether they wish to join a group. Of course, the motivation for change will need to come from the students as the group develops and as the students find they are important members with certain responsibilities to other group members and to themselves.

STEPS TO SUCCESS IN GROUP COUNSELING

The steps to success that are described here are organized in sequential order. The five steps are all important, but the first and last steps are most critical for effective groups.

Before You Start

As noted earlier, the educator about to undertake group counseling needs to obtain some support from a colleague who is experienced with counseling and who agrees to consult with the educator. In addition, the educator needs to plan the objectives for the group: just what do I hope to accomplish with this group? The colleague functioning as a consultant for the group can be of help even at this early stage by helping the educator scale back any unrealistic expectations for what could reasonably be accomplished in the group. Box 5.7 illustrates the advantage of clarity of leader expectation.

One important issue is that of group membership. Most writers on group counseling support the notion that group members will be voluntary participants and free to quit the group at any time. Therefore, the educator needs to address what will motivate a student to agree to join and remain in the group.

Often, students will be influenced by who else is to be in the group. The issue of group membership needs to be considered by the educator also. Homogeneous groups include members who have the same or similar problems and have the advantage of focusing the leader's thoughts and plans. Frequently, social skills groups and some behavioral groups will limit membership to only those students with similar concerns or areas of difficulty. Even homogeneous groups quickly show that each member is an individual and that no two

BOX 5.7. Clarity of Group Expectation

LACK OF CLARITY

At a meeting of eighth graders, Ms. T, the counseling leader, was listening carefully to the members. When Beckie asked whether she could bring pictures of her recent trip to Florida, Ms. T said, "O.K.," with some uncertainty.

Gradually, the "group" became a series of vacation descriptions as more and more members brought records of family vacations. Those members who had no photographs brought interesting pictures from travel magazines.

Ms. T experienced increasing frustration.

CLEARLY HELD LEADER GOALS

At a meeting of eighth grade students, Mr. T, the counseling leader, was asked whether one of the students could bring pictures from a recent vacation. Ms. T asked the group about the agreed-on purposes of the meetings. As the members reviewed their agree-on purposes with some prodding from Ms. T, it became clear that no mention had been made of members' family vacations.

Ms. T said, "Well, I guess this group wouldn't be the place for the pictures. What did you have in mind when you asked me if you could share them?"

Often the task is clearer when the leader has a mind set.

persons experience a problem in exactly the same way. In addition, with certain target groups, such as belligerent students, an entire group of similar individuals might seem too threatening or punishing for the leader. Heterogeneous groups may feature quite different members or even be formulated with a specific purpose in mind that will utilize the differences among group members. For example, three shy students could be combined with three quite outgoing, popular students into a single group so that the outgoing students would serve as role models and teach the shy students alternative behaviors, such as assertiveness.

The First Meeting

The first meeting is crucial because the group members will formulate their attitudes toward the group at this time. Of course, adolescents will seriously ogle the other members. Questions on each student's mind might be: Are these the students I want to spend time with? Do I belong here? What are we doing here?

The group facilitator can openly address the answer to the last question. Expectations for the group, its purposes, what is to be accomplished, and how many meetings and for how long need to be clear. Unless the group facilitator has structured a didactic in-

structional group, not likely in a counseling group, the first activity—
perhaps even prior to clarifying expectations—should be a warm-up
activity. An early impression can be formed that this group is going to
be fun, that the group will not be like another class (unless, of course,
that is the purpose of the group), and that the facilitator will be warm
and caring during the group meetings.

Members feeling apprehensive about the group, wondering how
they fit into the group now and how they will fit in later, and mentally
"sizing up" the group facilitator are to be expected. One of the first
issues for each member of a counseling group is that of individual
identity within the group (Yalom, 1985). The educator can help
members deal with many important issues during the first few meetings. Some authors have described the early meetings of a counseling
group as "milling around" and as the orientation stage.

Simultaneously with the clarifying of content, including the purposes of the group and what is to be accomplished during group
meetings, the group leader will need to begin to accomplish important process goals. The norms of a group are usually viewed as
established through collaboration between the leader and group
members. If the setting or the personal preferences of the facilitator
dictate certain limits on member behavior, then such norms, or rules
for operating within the group, need to be specified for the members.
Adherence to certain rules of conduct may be required if individuals
are to remain members.

In other cases, the facilitator can indicate as early as the first
meeting that the group will be asked to decide how to operate. These
early decisions take time and gradually help the group learn how to
participate in the group decision-making process. During the period
of establishing and enforcing group norms, the facilitator will want to
observe the group closely. How does group leadership emerge? Is
everyone participating? Do members interrupt each other? Do only
certain members get interrupted? There are a host of opportunities
for the attentive group leader to observe and to learn about the
members.

Some facilitators will choose to dictate certain norms—no violence
in the group, no talking about an absent member, no talking outside
of group about what happens at meetings, no smoking, and so on.
However, negotiable norms for some group leaders might include
such rules as no smoking, no talking outside of group about what
happens at meetings, what to do about members who come late, the
necessity to let a speaker finish what he/she is saying with no interruption, and so on. What some group facilitators consider nonnegotiable,
such as no smoking, other group leaders will see as advantageous to
negotiate with the group.

Two important factors influence the type of norms that will be set by the group and the amount of group responsibility in setting norms. These two factors have been described earlier in this chapter, namely, the theoretical preference of the leader and the purposes of the group. For example, behavioral groups may not spend very much time at all on establishing process norms but work hard to specify clearly the goals and expectations for group membership. Such a group might have individual members specify for the others exactly what behaviors they are in the group to work on changing. A Rogerian-style group could very easily have content goals such as learning about member potential or learning to make greater use of member strengths. Such rather vague content goals could not very easily be made any more concrete. The Rogerian group will take a great deal of responsibility for deciding how it will function and what the norms will be.

The purposes of the group also help the facilitator decide what needs to be covered at the first meeting. A learning group needs content, which can be introduced during the first meeting. Even when structured learning is a goal of the group, members will interact, will have some responsibility for how time is spent, and will participate in group decisions. Otherwise the "group" is just another task group or class and not a counseling group at all.

Getting to Work

As indicated earlier, different theoretical orientations influence when a group starts grappling with its task. However, for many counseling groups, the members have the responsibility for learning how to accomplish the work of the group. It is the members themselves who will help each other grow and change. After the facilitator has clarified the purposes fo the group, and when the group has begun to set norms for itself, the group can proceed to its central work. Although it is fairly common for some counseling groups to avoid the work stage, an effective group needs to get to work if only to avoid becoming an escape, a place to go to avoid the tasks of the school.

If the group facilitator, because of theoretical bent and purposes of the group, firmly points and directs the members to get to work, opportunity needs to be given for members to react to the leader's actions. When members avoid work or seem sluggish about buckling down to the task at hand, an effective leader can discuss this with members. Even in groups that have a strong emphasis on leader direction, members can take responsibility for their own actions, such as avoiding work.

In those cases in which group purpose and theoretical notions of the leader dictate, the group will assume almost all the responsibility for work. However, some groups never learn how to work together. Such a tendency can exist in groups in public schools. For example, a group of former chemical users will very likely have a day in which each group member just feels "blah" and doesn't choose to get very serious. However, groups of former users are most often highly motivated. Even more common is when the group accomplishes a lot and feels so good about itself that it prefers to relive the good day and hence avoid any new effort. The group leader can carefully attend to what the group is doing and attempt to facilitate the group's work. Many of the specific techniques and choices for the leader are discussed in the following chapter. However, for now, three examples follow.

At the third meeting of a highly structured group in a middle school, Jerry started off the session with the following: "I don't see what we're supposed to be doing. Why can't I go to music class?"

The facilitator, who thought that the purposes of the group had been thoroughly understood by all members, nevertheless responded by drawing all group members into a discussion of the expectations.

"Jerry, that's an interesting question. Let's see if we can help Jerry. Just what are we doing in this group while we're together?

At a junior high group led by a school psychologist, the members had been exploring together just how they could make new friends. During the third meeting, one member said to Sally: "I can see why you don't have any friends. No one likes your sister."

The facilitator decided that the opening offered by the statement to Sally was directly in line with the announced "work" of the group. Deciding to ignore the speaker, probably for a later time, the leader chose to focus the group concern on Sally.

"Sally, what do you think? Is it possible that some seventh graders avoid you because of your sister?"

Finally, at a high school group meeting dealing with recent personal loss, such as death or a divorce in the family, one member began to cry. The facilitator decided that the first response of the group to tears would likely be important to the continued sharing of personal information. She responded: "We can see that this is upsetting to you, Ginger. Let's all just be quiet and get in touch with our feelings for a moment."

Then the leader led a discussion in which the group, including Ginger, explored their feelings.

Getting Ready to End

All too frequently, the end of a counseling group coincides with the end of the school year or the vagaries of holiday schedules or even of changes in assignments. Suddenly it is June, or there is a new educator in the chair of an earlier one. Such predictable interruptions are not cause for abrupt termination to a counseling group. Any abrupt termination to a counseling group is to be avoided. The group leader has the responsibility to help the group anticipate its termination.

The educator needs to help the group work toward its own termination. As early as half way into the planned duration of the group, the facilitator can alert the members to the impending final date.

During a group session of high school students, one member stated, "I would like to pass today. I just don't feel like working on my contract."

LEADER: Well, Pat, we only have five more meetings, and we do have six other students who are working on changes. Are you sure you want to skip this week? We might not get back to you at our next meeting.

By the last two or three meetings, the facilitator will frequently be phrasing plans in terms of the impending date that signals the end of the group.

When a member expresses any thoughts or reactions to the upcoming end of the group, the facilitator would be wise to allow other students to express their reactions to the impending termination. It is expecting too much that all feelings will be explored or even shared at the last meeting. As members are given a chance to express themselves in terms of the upcoming final meeting, the group can take on more responsibility for the work to be done before terminating.

Groups are also good at slowing down in anticipation of "only three more meetings." In fact, educational settings are rife with students and professionals coasting the final days before a vacation. So one factor to be aware of is that as the leader prepares the group for closure, some members will decide to quit contributing, since there is so little time.

The facilitator can help the group "get back to work" just as getting to work was described in the previous section. The leader could say, for example, "Come on now. Our time is short and we have five more members who haven't had a chance to summarize their contracts yet."

The Last Meeting

Several important tasks can be considered by the facilitator in preparation for the last meeting. Of course, each group member needs time in the group to assess how far he/she has come and also time to summarize a reaction to or evaluation of the group to all the members. The group facilitator also has to estimate whether or not the timing of the group's closure is right for each member. Is this a good time and place to leave the member? Does a referral need to be made, since there will be no further meetings? Box 5.8 suggests items for the last meeting.

What transpires at the final meeting needs to include such individual assessment. If an individual was abruptly confronted, or perhaps chooses the last 5 minutes of the last meeting to announce, "I have been talking with my girlfriend about our killing ourselves," the facilitator must take appropriate action, in this case making a referral for the member to receive counseling.

Members need to think back about the life of the group and what they have accomplished as individuals and as a total group. Feelings of sadness and of relief that this is the last meeting can be expressed. Behavioral group leaders especially will lead the group into a discussion of how changes initiated in the group can be made to last and to transfer into other situations.

Every group member can be helped to express reactions to loss: the loss of people who had become important. A group of relative strangers in the beginning has now drawn close and has provided help for some members. The ending to friendships and to the group is a part of life and can be explored during the last meeting.

The final task for the facilitator at the last meeting is that of evaluation. One criticism of counseling, which applies especially to group counseling, is that any changes or good feelings don't last beyond the life of the counseling. All facilitators need to evaluate the

---

BOX 5.8. What to Cover the Last Meeting

1. Remind group that this is the last meeting.
2. Check with members to see if any issues are "hanging" and need to be addressed.
3. Members and leader provide individual summaries for each member about what has been accomplished and where each member is.
4. Activities allowing each member who wishes to state who has been of help and what each member has gained.
5. Leader stimulation of member attitudes toward leaving and feelings about ending of group.
6. Leader decision on whether to evaluate group, collect any data from members.
7. Leader announcement to members about when to expect follow-up contact; explanation of importance and purposes of follow-up.
8. Good-byes.

---

effectiveness of the group. Chapter 7 describes the importance of evaluation and suggests methods for evaluating counseling.

There is always a tension within a counselor between helping the client(s) and meeting the counselor's needs, such as feeling good about what is being accomplished. No place is this tension more acute than at the last meeting of a counseling group. How does a sensitive facilitator take time from the last meeting to evaluate? The answer is with planning and careful preparation. Evaluation is a must, as is described in Chapter 7.

Even though it was the end of the school year, Mr. Judd, the eighth grade Industrial Arts teacher, knew he needed to take time to let the group summarize their reactions to the meetings in which they had learned social skills, especially alternatives to the rude, loud behavior they had exhibited when the group began.

MR. JUDD: Guys, I want each of you to think back to our first meeting. Let's talk about what we have done in this group. What do you think you have learned?

Finally, the group leader needs to alert the members that they will be contacted again for a follow-up evaluation. Whether the follow-up is 30 days or 3 months, the facilitator needs to determine how each member will be reached. The importance of evaluation and how the results of the follow-up will be used can be clarified during the last group meeting. When members understand the need for evaluation and the importance of the evaluation to the facilitator, they will be likely to respond to follow-ups.

A follow-up can take the form of having the counselor send a brief questionnaire to the members of the group during the next term or semester. Mr. Judd alerted his social skills group that he would be doing this. Two months later he had the counselor distribute a short evaluation form. As was discussed in Chapter 3, a more exact evaluation might include ratings from other teachers of the targeted social skills. Were negative skills apparent? Were positive skills apparent? Did the teacher notice any change?

SUMMARY

There is an extreme need for group counseling services within educational settings. Frequently, such services are not offered at all or not offered with the frequency desired by a professional educator. It is likely that educators can successfully offer group counseling if they have a minimum of professional training, some experience, and/or the agreement of a trusted colleague to consult with them during the life of the group. Three selected theories were described with a focus on the expected outcomes for members of groups featuring each system. Goals or expected outcomes for members of counseling groups fall into attitude change, including increased self-awareness and self-acceptance, and behavior change.

The importance of obtaining support and consultation from a competent colleague was described. The need for careful determination of the goals for a counseling group was discussed. The goals of the group help to determine which students should be members, the type of activity to be used, and many of the functions and interventions of the group facilitator.

Specific issues in a group's development were discussed, such as the planning before the group starts, the first meeting, getting the group to work, and closing the group. The next chapter specifies just how a leader functions in a counseling group.

6

Group Counseling: Process and Content

This chapter is designed to provide some detailed direction for the school practitioner who is about to form a counseling group. Chapter 5 reviewed three selected theories and also outlined the steps to follow in beginning a counseling group. This chapter continues the step-by-step format where possible and, for the purposes of clarity, separates discussion of the process within group counseling from that of the content being discussed. Attention to the process of a group includes the nonverbal communication among the group members. Group process also includes who is not talking, who comes late, and which students seem to disagree with each other. There will be times when separating process from content issues seems arbitrary. In truth, the process of group counseling is heavily influenced by the purposes of the group and by the chosen role(s) the group leader is using to affect those purposes.

GROUP COUNSELING PROCESS

The reasons that a school practitioner might select group counseling include a desire to allow students to learn about their own actions and how to accommodate themselves to the actions of others. If the educator thought that a lecture or another class would accomplish the same purpose, then group counseling would not have been selected. The group leader will need to conceive a role for himself/herself that provides ample opportunity for the group members to learn about themselves and the consequences of their behaviors. Such learning needs to include learning from mistakes. The group counselor, as opposed to many teachers, can prepare himself/herself to watch the group stumble, take wrong turns, or even to explore blind alleys. Although this means that group counseling takes time, perhaps more time than an impatient practitioner thinks it should, it is from learning about such events that members may acquire understanding not likely to result from lectures or from most classes.

For example, learning to take responsibility for one's own behavior is often difficult to accomplish for many of the students judged to need group counseling the most. In group counseling, members learn to take responsibility by being given it. Many school practitioners, as they develop a role for themselves as group counselors, will need to practice patience and learn to allow time for the group to explore and to make mistakes.

For example, in a junior high school, an assistant principal leading his first counseling group was surprised to learn that one of the group members was systematically borrowing money from each of the other group members. Apparently this member was not paying anyone back and using the earlier successful loans as "collateral" for making new ones.

"Oh come on. Everyone else in the group has loaned me money. Aren't you as much a part of the group as they are?" asked the member when a student refused him, apparently for the first time.

Rather than bring up the issue of borrowing in group, the assistant principal asked instead, "How have things been going outside of group? Anything to report?"

Not too surprisingly, one of the members complained about loaning money and not getting repaid. The assistant principal decided to help the group "process" what had happened. This allowed the assistant principal to respond to the "charges" from each of the aggrieved group members and to draw out the "offending" group member. Rather than interacting with the student from his authority role, the assistant principal was sincere in his effort to creat a new role as a group counselor and to discontinue his regular behaviors as the assistant principal.

The reader can predict the reactions of the group members if the principal had lectured the group or got on the case of the borrower. By taking responsibility, the group leader would have framed the issue in terms of what "ought" to be. Instead, as the members discovered that several of them had been duped, the discussion was directed toward learning from what had happened and, even more important, toward setting norms for what it meant to be a member in good standing of this group. The members discussed what behaviors they would find acceptable for "our" group.

Processing comments and interventions by a group leader are those that are designed to have individuals or all group members learn from what has been allowed to happen. The leader focuses the group, has to bring the group back to processing, and helps the group learn from the discussion.

The helpful elements in group psychotherapy have been described by Yalom (1985). Although one of these, interpersonal learning, was described in Chapter 5, 10 of Yalom's "curative factors" from group psychotherapy are listed in Box 6.1.

Although a group counseling leader might value altruism or might desire instillation of hope for particular members of a counseling group, effective groups are those in which the "curative factors" develop from the members. In fact, it is not likely, even in a very repressive educational climate, that the factors described in Box 6.1 can be imposed.

BOX 6.1. Helpful Elements of Group Psychotherapy

Ten "curative factors" (Yalom, 1985) are listed below. Although expressly described for psychotherapy, these elements are also found in counseling groups.

1. Instillation of hope results from the support individual members experience as they learn that other members and the group leader are willing to help them.

2. Universality occurs as individual members learn that other people also suffer from some of the same conflicts and feelings as they do.

3. Imparting of information is especially helpful as other group members share advice and their own experiences.

4. Altruism occurs as individuals who were formerly wrapped up in their own difficulties begin to focus on others and try to help them succeed.

5. Development of socializing techniques seems especially applicable to the school age group member, although it is worth noting that Yalom describes a process that takes the adult members of his groups months to accomplish.

6. Imitative behavior almost always occurs in a successful group. As members allow other group members to become important to them, they often emulate some of the person's behavior.

7. Interpersonal learning occurs as members exchange views and discuss their reactions to each other's behavior over the time of the group.

8. Group cohesiveness is the close feeling developed among the members in successful groups.

9. Catharsis occurs as members express their feelings in the safety of the group.

10. Existential factors involve the realization by members that they are responsible for their own behavior.

For example, it is our experience that trust in a group develops at the speed of the least trusting member. Even when one or two members of a group "insist" that all members hurry up and start trusting each other, complete trust among group members occurs at the speed of the least trusting member. This characteristic of trust is described here to illustrate the impossibility of dictating group climate. The leader in a counseling group cannot insist on a certain attitude or atmosphere within the group no matter how much he/she wishes it. Group climate has to evolve.

Processing provides a vehicle for the group leader to understand what group members are thinking, how they are perceiving what is happening in the group, and just where certain individuals see themselves within the group. A selected listing of leader statements that can be used in processing will illustrate the variety of techniques that are available.

PROCESS SKILLS BY LEADERS

A list of suggested skills for leaders to initiate group processing is found in Box 6.2.

Direct Questions

Questions to one group member may include:
"Ted, what seems to be happening in the group right now?"
"Jerry, is the group helping you right now?"
In both cases, the leader can redirect any statements of blame or put-down statements toward the group in general. Usually processing provides a time when the entire group can participate.
Other direct questions include:
"Let me ask the group if you are satisfied with our progress so far."
"Can someone tell me just what the group is so excited about?"
"What are we going to do about members who miss group?"

BOX 6.2. Leader Process Skills

1. *Direct questions:* questions to individual group members and to the entire group about the group.
2. *Focusing comments:* statements that direct members to respond about how the group is functioning.
3. *Process comments:* statements in which the leader indicates how he/she believes the group is functioning or that show that the leader wishes feedback from members about how the group is functioning.

Focusing Comments

"I'd like to return to Mary. It seems we didn't finish with you. We just drifted into another topic. Where are you right now, Mary?"

"It seems we sometimes don't finish a topic but just drift into a new one. Does anyone think we just did that again?"

"Today, I'd like to start the meeting by discussing how we are doing. Does it seem as though we've accomplished anything so far?"

Process Comments

For lack of a better word, just asking the group to process previous events or to share current reactions may work.

"Let's look at what is happening right now."

"Is anyone willing to tell us what you are feeling right now?"

"This silence may be a good time for us to process."

"Where are we?"

In a demonstration group that was a part of a counseling practicum in group counseling, the student leader said, "Let's process."

The group responded with, "Oh, no. We hate that. Let's not."

The group leader reported in supervision seminar that he guessed his group wouldn't be processing any more because of the comments from the group. The supervisor disagreed.

Using Process Skills

As the practitioner begins to meet with groups of students, it is important to remember the necessity of allowing time, and even teaching students, to process. There is no substitute for the group members sharing their different perceptions; for learning that one member's exciting group is another member's boring day; that members disagree about what is helpful; that people differ as to how fast is enough. Processing offers the means for group members to learn about themselves as individuals and about themselves as members of a group.

Although groups with elementary students will differ from those with older students, the group facilitator can work with members to recognize when group process issues are being discussed. For example, Ms. Brown asked her group of fourth graders to consider: "How are we behaving differently in this group from the way most of us behave in class?"

Early in the life of the group, the leader can initiate group discussion about what is happening between and among group members. Some groups will start with the leader repeating what the expectations are for each group member, as was already covered in the individual screening interviews discussed in the previous chapter. Other groups will start with the leader stating, for the first time, just what the purposes of the group are and what will be expected of each member. Still other groups may start with, "What would you like to do in this group?" Many educational settings would not tolerate an extended period of such discussion of what members would like to do, given the need to accommodate other demands such as required courses and pressures from parents to keep students involved in academics.

With any counseling group, however, members need time to assimilate and to react to what they are experiencing. A group begins to assume responsibility for itself when it makes a change in a rule or when it decides on a rule and then adheres to this self-imposed regulation. Assuming responsibility begins with having some responsibility, as in the conduct of the group.

Even at early meetings, the leader can lead a session toward closure, 10 or 15 minutes before the designated end, by asking the group members to summarize what has happened. Such group processing allows the leader to identify different perceptions and to begin to judge the perceptiveness of group members.

Group leaders in our experience have singled out individuals for this task.

"Mindy, would you summarize what you think has happened in group today?"

However, this practice of calling on an individual tends to pressure group members and may disallow the sharing of group perceptions about what is happening. As members exchange perceptions of and reactions to each meeting, greater understanding and sharing among members occur.

At times a leader may wish to begin a session with a summary of the previous meeting or even of all the meetings so far. As long as there is no rush and each individual is allowed to participate, this method is useful to members. In fact, beginning a session with a discussion of process may lead naturally to clarification of goals. Note how the leader in the following example seeks to get a commitment (goals) from the group members.

"So it sounds like I wasn't the only one who wished Mary and Pete had had some time last meeting to finish their discussion. What if this time one of you ask Pete and Mary what they are thinking during our meeting today. Are you willing to do that?"

At later meetings, the leader can process during the meeting rather than only at the end or the beginning. As members learn to discriminate between group work and processing about group work, they will become adept at moving between the two. However, students in graduate classes on group counseling are not always able to discriminate between processing and discussing, so expecting younger students to do so may be unrealistic.

When asked to process by the group leader, one group responded with a member asking, "Did anyone see the movie on HBO last night?" This statement distracted the group from processing.

Assertive behavior by a group leader is called for if a group drifts off a topic or if the group is actively resisting processing. Firm statements about the importance of discussing what is happening or calm repetition of a request are examples of such assertiveness.

Halfway through a semester, a group session of high school students ended with an international student tearfully sharing her loneliness and her difficulty making friends in the United States. When the leader asked for processing of "What happened last week, especially at the end of our session?," no one in the group addressed the content of the message of the international student. Instead, the group playfully bantered about upcoming tests and papers.

The group leader was confident that the members could successfully handle their discomfort with Khalil's tears from the week before. So the leader asked again, "What are your reactions to Khalil stating how hard it was for her to make friends here in Caucasian High?"

It is especially important for the group leader to develop the ability to discriminate between processing and other discussions within the counseling group. It is unlikely that a group will be able to learn when they are processing and when they are not if the leader has trouble discriminating between the two. Through purposeful attending to discussion, the practitioner can practice the discrimination of content from the process going on in a group. In addition, references such as George and Dustin (1988) and those in Appendix B are recommended for further reading.

Statements requesting group processing, even if taken from the list provided in this chapter (see Box 6.2), do not automatically result in a group's processing.

Ms. Amels was an experienced teacher who decided to form a counseling group from among her eighth grade science students who were having difficulty in her classes. She carefully thought through her goals and expectations for the group before soliciting students to participate. At the close of the second session, Ms. Amels asked the students, "Are you satisfied with our progress so far?"

The students were silent. Ms. Amels asked, "Don't any of you have an opinion?"

The silent students fidgeted.

"All right, I'm going to send you all back to class if one of you doesn't respond."

The reader doesn't need further description of how the teacher reverted to her authority role. Another response might have been to ask the students about their silence.

"You're all pretty quiet. I wonder what the silence means."

There is no question that if the teacher can wait long enough, a student will respond, even if only with the question, "What do you mean?"

Such an opening allows the teacher to gently ask the group again to look at its own behavior, in this case the silence in response to the question, "Are you satisfied with our progress [in group] so far?"

PRACTICAL LEADER TECHNIQUES

Although professional education vacillates between periods stressing specific techniques and periods deriding "cookbook" education, a select list of group leader techniques is offered. Some of the techniques were included in the Addendum to Chapter 3, "Skills for Interviewers." However, the use of the techniques differs in a group. In addition, different theoretical orientations would feature different usage from the list that follows. The purpose of the group will also influence certain leader roles leading to different emphases in the use of the listed techniques.

Box 6.3 lists the techniques described in this section with a brief definition for each.

Responses to Feelings

There are several techniques that can facilitate processing since they are directed at the feelings of members of the group.

Acknowledging Feelings

Sometimes in their eagerness to facilitate group processing, beginning group leaders will rush right by the expressed feelings of a member. Just an acknowledgment can be very important to the person expressing the feeling. It is a sure sign that the leader has heard and recognized the feeling. Examples are as varied as there are different leadership styles.

BOX 6.3. Practical Leader Techniques Addressing Affect

---

1. *Acknowledging feelings expressed by members:* a statement that relates to a feeling just stated by a member.
2. *Restating the feeling:* a word-for-word repetition of a member statement that includes an expressed feeling.
3. *Paraphrase of feelings:* a shortened version of a member statement that uses a synonym for the feeling or that repeats the feeling.
4. *Adding to feelings:* a leader statement that accentuates a feeling of a member or the entire group. Sometimes questions can add to the expression of feelings by group members.
5. *Asking for feelings:* questions about feelings directed at individual members or at the entire group.
6. *Drawing in other members:* asking for other members to respond to feelings expressed by a group member.
7. *Leader self-disclosure:* by expressing their own current feelings, group leaders can help the group react to feelings and express their own feelings.

LEADER: I bet you did.
LEADER: Yes, we can see that.
LEADER: Will someone respond to Mary's excitement?

Restating the Feeling

Although subject to overuse, one method of responding to feelings is for the leader to restate the expressed feeling. In the event the leader has misperceived the emotion, restatement serves to clear up misunderstanding, since the speaker's response will almost always be to correct the mistake by reexpressing the feeling. In other cases, accurate restatement by the leader can serve to show group members that feelings are worth talking about and that they are a part of group processing. Two examples of restatement follow.

GROUP MEMBER: I just am so happy to see you all. It's surprising to me how important this group has become in just 2 short weeks.
LEADER: You're really happy to see us and surprised at the same time.
GROUP MEMBER: I almost didn't come to group today. I just really feel down.
LEADER: You are really down and almost didn't come to group.

The drawback to a word-for-word restating of feelings is that the technique is noticeable to the student. In fact, out of exasperation, a student might say, "That's just what I said!" Another skill that overcomes the limitation of exact repetition is paraphrasing.

Paraphrase of Feelings

Usually a shortened version of what has been expressed, a paraphrase sounds more natural than word-for-word repetition or restatement. Such shortened versions, if they include the feeling that was expressed by the speaker, are excellent means of responding to feelings and help the group keep abreast or aware of feelings as the members process. Three examples follow (for more complete exercises and examples, the reader is referred to Egan, 1976, or Colangelo, Dustin, & Foxley, 1982).

GROUP MEMBER: So I just didn't know what to say, I was stunned. I finally blurted out something, and left there as fast as I could.
LEADER: It really threw you.

GROUP MEMBER: I almost didn't come to school today. I laid around the house and purposely missed the bus. That's why I was late. I just felt down and didn't think I could face you all.
LEADER: It was hard to think about facing us when you were so down.

GROUP MEMBER: I'm just not sure that my behavior is so bad. Sometimes I don't even think I belong in this group. All the kids are just as bad as me.
LEADER: You're not sure you belong in this group.

Adding to Feelings

Since the leader is trying to help the group understand what is happening in the group and to begin to take responsibility for what occurs during the group sessions, the feelings of individual members are relevant during processing. At times, feelings will remain just below the surface and will not be directly expressed. Therefore, the leader can add to the quality of communication during processing by focusing on such feelings and encouraging the members to react to and to acknowledge the feelings. For example:

LEADER: I notice that you all started talking about papers you have due when I asked you to process what happened at the end of last group, when Khalil expressed how lonely she was in America. Could it be that it was hard for you to talk about?

It is important that a leader facilitate the group's discussion of feelings rather than sound accusatory or indicate blame in some way.

Groups can learn to discuss feelings and can develop the capacity to respond to member feelings without depending on the leader. In another example:

GROUP MEMBER: I don't know what to do. Every week I just promise to keep the contract, and then at the next meeting, I haven't done anything.
LEADER: Could it be that you find it hard to face the need to change?

For a final example:

LEADER: Let's process.
GROUP MEMBERS: Oh, no. We hate that. Not again.
LEADER: Why is it so hard to talk about what we are doing in the group?

It is possible to add to the expression of feelings by asking about feelings, which leads to another method of responding to emotions when they are raised in the group.

Asking for Feelings

With this technique, the leader does not take the responsibility of specifically labeling or repeating expressed feelings or of accurately "adding to" feelings. Asking for feelings is a method of focusing, just as asking for processing was described as one method of focusing the group's attention on process.

LEADER: No one is saying it, but I sense some resentment in the group. Am I right?
LEADER: Who can tell me how you are feeling right now?
LEADER: Will someone tell me how they feel about this group?

When asking for feelings, the group leader is signaling to group members that the group is a place in which feelings will be listened to and will be taken seriously. The group leader asks for feelings in order to teach the members to recognize and to express their feelings in the group.

Drawing in Other Members

Even when a member has expressed a feeling, the leader may wish to encourage other members to react or even to express the same feeling. Some of the earlier responses on this list feature the leader responding to feelings. But group processing was not defined in this chapter as a leader's view of what is happening in the group. It is ultimately necessary to facilitate an all-member discussion about the group.

Examples of drawing in other members regarding expressed feelings include the following:

GROUP MEMBER: I just feel stifled. This group just sits and looks at each other and waits for you to talk.
LEADER: How about someone else? Does anyone else feel the same way?

GROUP MEMBER: I almost didn't come today. I just couldn't think about facing this group.
LEADER: Is she the only one who has felt like this? Do any of you ever dread coming to group?

LEADER: Let's process.
GROUP MEMBER: Let's not. I hate this.
LEADER: Is Mark the only one who feels this way?

There are, potentially, many specific feelings that might be expressed or hinted at in a group. The reader should see these examples as getting at only three: feeling stifled, dread, and avoidance or hesitancy. Group leaders can respond to feelings experienced simultaneously by several members as well as to those of individuals. An example of acknowledging such feelings might be:

LEADER: It sounds as though the whole group is impatient to get some specific activities started.

An example of adding to commonly experienced feelings might be:

LEADER: So several of you have lots of reasons for coming late to each meeting. I wonder if coming late is a sign of something else. Could it be that you guys don't want to be in this group?

In other words, asking for group feelings can draw several members into the discussion.

There is more to processing than eliciting member feelings about what is happening in the group, although member feelings are crucial to effective group processing. However, increased understanding is the primary purpose of group processing. Members are to learn about themselves, about the impact of their behavior on other group members, and that the accomplishments of the group are influenced by how the group spends its time. Box 6.4 describes some typical incidents from group counseling and indicates how a leader might use these techniques to respond.

Leader Self-Disclosure

There is quite a variance among writers in group psychotherapy about how much leader self-disclosure is optimal. Predictably, behavioral group leaders focus quite sharply on the content of the group, that is, each member's behavior change, and therefore use self-disclosure only sparingly. Adlerian and Rogerian leaders often see leader self-disclosure as susceptible to overuse and recommend caution. What are some of the considerations that might influence effective leader self-disclosure?

First of all, leader self-disclosure is the expression of any opinion, attitude, or feeling by the leader. Self-disclosure does not have to be from deep, dark reaches of a psyche. Any opinion is viewed as self-disclosure (Dustin & Curran, 1985). An example is:

LEADER: I think this is an attractive room we have to meet in.

BOX 6.4. Group Situations and Possible Leader Responses

1. *Member silence.* Often pauses in conversation seem much longer to a leader than they actually are. During the silence the leader can:
   a. Scan the group. What are members communicating nonverbally?
   b. Think about what preceded the silence. Did the leader just speak? Could the members be thinking?

2. *Member resistance.* Although one person's interpretation that a group is resisting may be another's thought that the group is developing to a new stage (such as conflict stage), a leader can help the group through such periods.
   a. Let all members talk, being careful that one or two members don't monopolize and don't try to speak for all group members.
   b. Focus on feelings and try to get members to express their feelings.
   c. Monitor leader defensiveness. When the leader finds himself/herself becoming defensive, often a simple "I" statement will clear the air.

3. *Expressions of hostility.* The leader needs to point out to the group any ground rules that have been negotiated and then help the group decide how to respond.
   a. The leader can support the member who is the target of hostility, see if the member is listening, and see if the member wishes to respond. Point out to the group if an attack is underway.
   b. Reflect feelings of anger as they are expressed.

Another is:

LEADER: I hope all of you will make yourselves comfortable here in the meeting room.

A final example is:

LEADER: I know I never went that far on a date when I was in ninth grade.

Self-disclosure is a means for the leader to express his/her own opinions and feelings and to allow the group to get to know the leader as a person.

An obvious caution about leader self-disclosure is overuse. If the leader repeatedly expresses feelings during the group, then the leader runs the risk of meeting his/her own needs at the expense of member needs. The reader may be able to recall a counselor or teacher, if not a group counselor, who overused self-disclosure by using lengthy reminiscences about "the great war" or "my senior prom." All too often these "self-disclosures" are seen by the listener as boring or irrelevant.

Ivey and Gluckstern (1976) have done all educators a service by describing effective self-disclosure as always including an element of checking out the self-disclosure—that is, asking the listeners, in this case the group, whether they got the point or whether there seemed to be a point to the self-disclosure. Such advice is worth memorizing. Two examples of leader self-disclosure follow.

GROUP MEMBER: So I just can't stand when we come to the part of the group where you say, "Let's process."
LEADER: I know sometimes I feel in faculty meetings, "Here we go again." I wonder will we ever get out of this.

At the meeting after Khalil stated her difficulties making friends in the United States, the leader stated, "I am really bothered that none of you responded when Khalil opened up her feelings of aloneness. I'm afraid that she will only feel more lonely."

INVOLVING STUDENTS IN PROCESSING

Earlier in this chapter, detailed attention was given to methods a group counselor might use to facilitate group processing. The reader is invited to review that section.

Nevertheless, there are certain specific methods a leader can use to accomplish processing by the group. For example, by stating his/her own current feelings, a group leader can signal to the group that feeling statements are legitimate. At other times, such self-disclosure might help the leader indicate to the group that time spent processing what had happened in group was important.

LEADER: I can tell that this is not easy for you. Several of you have been quiet. But I think that it is important for the group to spend time looking at itself. I hope you'll keep trying to answer my question, "What are your reactions to what has happened in group so far?"

Box 6.5 lists an example of an observation sheet that a group counselor could have filled in by an observer, either a student, probably a member of the group, or a colleague. In cases where group members agree, the leader may tape record sections of the group and then use the observation sheet to count specific techniques.

THE CONTENT OF GROUP COUNSELING

The "content" of a group is the subject(s) under discussion. Inexperienced group leaders usually get caught up in the content at the expense of noticing such important process elements as who is silent,

BOX 6.5. Observation Sheet of Leader Skills

Techniques	Tally		
Direct questions			
Questions about feelings			
Questions directed at the whole group			
Process comments			
Paraphrase			
Paraphrase of feeling			
Self-disclosure			
Did leader check it out?			

who seems bored, and so on. Nevertheless, groups do talk about something, and we turn now to some practical leader techniques designed to facilitate member understanding of group content. Box 6.6 lists the techniques suggested here for responding to member content.

Similar techniques used in individual counseling were discussed in Chapter 4. The labels for the techniques are not as important as the fact that effective counseling utilizes these techniques in individual and group settings.

Active Listening

The leader serves as a model for members by carefully listening to the speaker. Alert facial expression, smiles, head nods, as well as other nonverbal behaviors are important elements of active listening. Leaders with younger group members will no doubt have to spend considerable energy getting the norm of listening established in the group.

Questions

Just as with teaching, a common and effective way to respond to content is by asking questions. Questions serve to show a speaker that the questioner is interested, cares about the topic, and is following. Sometimes direct, closed questions can slow an eager speaker down. Such questions may also serve to focus on only a part of what the speaker is discussing.

LEADER: Gerry, what did you say had happened right before algebra class?

LEADER: Jim, tell us again how you felt when you were kicked out of the lunch room.

BOX 6.6. Techniques Used to Respond to Content

1. Active listening. Leader listening to members and communicating interest and caring nonverbally
2. Questions about what is being said.
3. Restatement. Word-for-word repetition by leader of member statement.
4. Paraphrase. Leader responds to a member statement with a shortened version that accurately captures the meaning of the member.
5. Summary. A paraphrase over an extended period of time, which may include statements by more than one member.

Open questions, defined earlier, may prove effective when the leader wishes to draw out a speaker or to show the group that one way of responding to a speaker is by asking questions.

LEADER: Jim, why do you suppose you were the only person kicked off the school bus?
LEADER: How did you feel then, Judy?

Restatement

This technique can be just as effective when the focus is content as when emotion is part of the statement. Restating content helps the entire group follow the speaker, can show a speaker whether the group is understanding, and is especially useful when important negotiations are being discussed.

LEADER: So you will weigh in twice before our next meeting, and you'll tell us just how much you lose or gain. Did I get that right?

Paraphrases

Discussed earlier in techniques of individual counseling and also as a process technique in group counseling, paraphrasing is still a helpful response when the focus is content. Shortened versions of what the speaker says help both listener and speaker track the communication during a conversation and can result in increased understanding. It is one thing to say, "I understand." It is another to show such understanding by repeating back a shortened version of what a speaker just said.

GROUP MEMBER: It was really hard for me to leave chorus this period to come to our group. It's only 3 days till our performance, and I hated to miss class.
LEADER: It was hard for you to miss music this period.

Summaries

A paraphrase that includes content raised at an earlier session can be considered a summary. A group leader can focus the group and can steer the conversation by summarizing something that was stated earlier. In group counseling, it is important to check out the accuracy of a summary. Since the group leader creates a role with a different authority structure from that of a teacher, it seems sensible to remember to end a summary by checking it out with the group.

"What do you think about what I just said?"

"Is that about how you remember our last meeting?"

Usually it will not be as important for a group to agree with the leader's perception—summary—as it will for the group to discuss and share reactions to what was said or to what actually happened.

Content of behavioral groups will usually include a series of individual progress reports as members are engaged in individual change programs. It can be especially effective as a method for a leader to keep the group on task or to show what remains to be done in the remaining time.

LEADER: So we haven't heard from Roger or Sue yet, and we only have 15 minutes left.

Developing the skill of using summaries effectively can be of use to leaders with any theoretical orientation. The practical techniques become smoother and more natural as they are used. In every case, no one technique is the only effective one. Group leaders develop a repertoire and become adept at selecting techniques as they develop experience and learn the effects of techniques in certain situations.

The reader can see that a number of key techniques are used in both individual and group counseling. In addition, many of the important skills can help members understand content and also learn about group process. By placing examples in several different places in this text, we hoped to show different examples of the techniques when they are used for different purposes.

CONTENT COMMON TO MANY GROUPS

Although groups will be formed for many purposes, certain key content will be expected with groups of school-age students. Box 6.7 lists some of the topics often addressed in group counseling.

There will be some uncertainty and some negative feelings expressed early in the group. These comments can be predicted, especially until group members feel secure about the purposes of the group and about their place in the group.

For example, comments such as the following are quite common:

"I don't know what I'm doing in here. I sure don't belong with you guys."

"Now what are we supposed to be doing in here again?"

BOX 6.7. Common Topics in Group Counseling

Elementary students
    Individual issues: role in group; relationship with friends
    Reasons for group: why individual is member
    Attitudes towards others: subgroups in school; parents/siblings
    Discussion of junior high

Middle school students
    Relationships with friends
    Attitude toward opposite sex
    Reasons for group: whether other students can join
    Teachers, school, need for homework
    Parents

Senior high students
    Relationships with peers
    Teachers, school, homework
    Work
    Parents
    Relationships with opposite sex
    Future plans: doubts; preparation for vocation/future education

As the group leader patiently explains the purposes of the group again, members will often center their remarks around their personal reactions to the content. For example, a group on study skills can be expected to dwell on teachers: on their unfairness, their tendency to expect too much homework, and their habit of picking favorites. The content of these remarks can best be understood as masking the individual members' concern about their own academic progress.

A group selected for the purpose of social skill development can, of course, expect quite a period of denial as the self-conscious adolescents or preadolescents demonstrate that they have no need for any additional social development, because of course, they are "cool" or have very active social lives. The facilitator who gets caught up in this content, especially caught up enough to start debating with individuals that "Yes, you do too need to develop these skills," is unnecessarily going to make it harder for the group members. Process comments, along with acceptance of member denial, can help the group progress through this early stage and get on with the "work" of the group, accomplishing group goals.

A part-time teacher in a middle school initiated a group for sixth grade boys who needed to develop some social skills. After soliciting recommendations from several teachers, the staff member, Ms. Kline, met with the boys who were recommended. After the boys who were interested volunteered, and after Ms. Kline decided that she could handle only seven boys in this first group attempt, the meetings were scheduled.

As might be expected, the first meeting was unruly and quite discouraging for Ms. Kline. Although the boys were polite enough when she repeated the reasons for the group and went over her expectations for group membership, whenever asked to react to her remarks or when asked what was on their minds about making friends, the boys talked about television programs, the upcoming sixth grade track meet, and other seemingly nonrelated topics.

After expressing her discouragement to the school psychologist, Ms. Kline followed his advice and held another meeting. This time the boys spent less time off the subject but frequently asked her to repeat why they were meeting and just what they were supposed to do. Often, the questions came too fast to answer, and Ms. Kline noticed that the boys didn't always listen to her answers. Finally, instead of dealing literally with the content of each question, Ms. Kline asked, "Are some of you guys worried about being in this group, maybe about what your friends will think about your being here?"

As mentioned earlier, at times content takes a back seat as the facilitator focuses on the process in the group. By careful listening, group facilitators can keep in touch with members and their concerns. However, discussion of content can be a mask for client concerns and underlying doubts. With experience, the educator can help the group to address the underlying issues. Mastering the challenge of dealing with both content and process issues lies at the heart of successful group counseling.

7

Evaluating the Effectiveness of Counseling

Counseling done by school practitioners can involve short periods of contact with students or longer, more intensive forms of intervention. Whatever the duration and outcome of involvement with students, evaluating the effects of the professional's efforts is recommended. Writers on the topic of evaluating counseling mention the importance of documenting the efforts that went into producing change as well as the impact of services on the student as well as the service provider.

Both the process and products of counseling with the individual student can be evaluated, as we will soon see; in addition to an investigation of the counseling experience, the professional can monitor the broader program of counseling services made available in the school. Monitoring how such services are provided, which students end up benefiting from such services, and how acceptable such services are to parents can be part of the evaluation of counseling programs. In this chapter, we review important information on how counseling can be evaluated at the client and at program levels. Discussion is provided of an additional level of assessment, that of soliciting perceived needs of parents, educators, and professionals for counseling services.

THE PROCESS AND PRODUCTS OF COUNSELING

Writers who describe strategies for evaluation in school programs have emphasized the importance of focusing on the full extent of services being provided in every facet of delivery to children. Terms that are used to describe the various components of evaluation are formative evaluation and summative evaluation. These terms were developed as labels for use during consideration of both the process and outcomes of an intervention effort.

Formative evaluation in counseling, for example, can serve the professional by first documenting which services were provided in which sequence, which professionals and clients were involved in each aspect of those services, and whether any component of the goals and objectives was not implemented. Formative evaluation, if conducted to accomplish such documentation, can provide the professional with a clear picture of the effectiveness of counseling interventions.

Why is such documentation valuable? From experience, most school practitioners realize that in the hustle and bustle of working with children, the details involved are remembered for only brief periods of time. Students demand our attention, and we typically respond in an immediate or short-term fashion. After all, if we wait too long to begin interventions with children, their needs can change. So formative evaluation offers the professional a set of strategies or questions to consider that will provide necessary documentation to account for the time and energies devoted to counseling.

Formative evaluation is more than basic record keeping or documentation. Formative evaluation is an appropriate activity only when the practitioner has prepared for the counseling experience by setting goals and objectives for what will be accomplished, provided timelines for the delivery of such services, and considered how the strategies and techniques that will applied during counseling will be selected and assessed (see Box 7.1). For example, the practitioner wanting to work with a child can prepare for formative evaluation by setting, at the beginning of contact, limits and priorities on what should be accomplished during involvement with the student. Goals and objectives are not, as might be expected, set in concrete but are subject to change with shifts in circumstances or priorities on either the client's or the professional's part. The planning that goes into delivering services, including identification of materials, scheduling of times for encounters, contacting parents to fill them in on experiences, or setting up schedules for groups of students to participate, all will enter into the formative evaluation process. As events unfold, the professional can review what had been expected to occur, make adjustments as necessary to plans, and prepare for future components of the counseling endeavor. As we recommend in earlier chapters, a colleague can be consulted on a regular basis to get feedback on what is being planned and accomplished.

In one school program, the school counselor had developed a system that worked well over the years for what we have called formative evaluation. Every referral for services was taken orally as

BOX 7.1. The Process of Individual Counseling

1. Agreement between the student and the practitioner to work together (may take several contacts before the student commits to action).
2. The Who, What, When, and Where of counseling. Actions to be taken by the student can be specified so that both parties (student and practitioner) know what actions will be taken, at what time, and in what location.
3. Plans for action can be modified. All modifications, however, should be documented.
4. Unplanned events or actions can become part of the evaluation of process examination, simply for documentation or evaluation.
5. The goal of process evaluation is to insure accountability of all parties. A secondary consequence is establishing documentation regarding your involvement.

well as in writing. The counselor took extensive notes every time a teacher, parent, or student requested services. These notes, after additional contact with the client and family, were considered when the counselor worked with the student to agree on goals.

In another district, a teacher who counseled one or two students a year had a similar system of keeping track of what had been discussed or done with the student. The teacher was aware that, given the limited time spent in counseling, he could easily forget exactly what had been said and done with students seeking advice or attention. Agreements, or contracts, between both parties were entered into notes that he maintained in his home office.

Goals that emerge from initial discussions can become part of the contract between the student and the practitioner. The contract can include a listing of all expected activities that will address goals and objectives, provide a timeline within which the services will be delivered (2 weeks, an entire academic semester, a school year), and furnish additional information on what the student and practitioner will gain when the contract is completed.

The counselor described above kept a file on each student served and included the contract to aid in eventual documentation of activities. Into that file went a brief note that provided information on all telephone and face-to-face encounters that the counselor had with the client. Information would be included, for example, on what the student said during sessions or over the telephone, activities during group or individual counseling sessions that reflected goals and objectives, and other information that appeared relevant at the time. On a regular basis, the counselor would review what was in the file and eliminate all information that was not directly related to efforts to evaluate process or products.

As has been noted, timelines, activities, and eventual outcomes are subject to negotiation. When changes occur in agreements or contracts, notes become a point of reference for the practitioner and the student. In the example above, the counselor, on a biweekly basis, would send notes to the student providing a very brief summary of progress. Copies of the notes went into the folder kept on each student by the counselor. Using this process, the counselor was confident that relatively little information centering on client contact escaped becoming documented. Access to the folder was restricted to the counselor, the student, and other parties with a legal right to access.

A social worker in a different school district followed similar procedures. In addition, she rated both her own and the client's performance every month in accomplishing projected activities. Although her intent was not to provide outcome data on actual changes in client behavior, the social worker did want to have some form of evidence on the effort being put into the counseling activities. Thus, on a regular basis, the practitioner would take note of how much time and energy she devoted to working with the student individually or in a group and similarly noted effort that the student appeared to be putting into all scheduled or unscheduled activities. Rating scales that focus on the process of counseling can be developed to reflect the priorities of the individual professional and school program. Keep in mind, however, that evaluation forms used in the formative component will serve to document that events are occurring as planned to address goals and objectives.

George and Cristiani (1986) have written about the difficulty that many professionals have in conceptualizing or defining what is meant by the process of counseling. When we think about producing changes in a student's decision-making or problem-solving skills, we can project ahead about how the student could behave to exemplify better decision-making or problem-solving skills. However, what process events are relevant to producing changes? Counseling as a field of endeavor has no common set of strategies that will lead the professional toward a specific objective. Instead, a variety of theories and philosophies and methods have dictated progress in the profession. Thus, rather than focusing on rigorous definitions of process events, we choose to emphasize the importance of defining a plan of action that can be maintained, through monitoring and feedback, until expected outcomes can be evaluated.

The practitioner has the option, of course, of defining process events in such a way that they can be assessed. For example, a school teacher working with students in a group counseling activity can develop a form or scale to note or rate the interactions that occur among participants. A number of rating scales do exist by which communication flow can be noted and interpreted. For example, Stone (1980) has reported on some research in which communication during counseling exchanges was assessed. Ehly, Dustin, and Bratton (1983) have reported on an additional system that can be used to provide information on the focus and use of specific communication techniques during exchanges between the service provider and the client.

Ms. Brown, a third grade teacher, was about to conduct a series of group meetings for children in both third grade classrooms who had recently been faced with a separation or divorce of their parents. As she made preparations for her first meeting with the group, Ms. Brown decided to place, during the meeting, a 5" × 8" card in her lap so that she could tally each time any child talked (the children's initials were on the card). After the first meeting, Ms. Brown noted that two of the children had only talked once. She realized that she could have failed to tally some remarks from the children, but the tallies for the two children stood out because the other children had made 10 or more remarks.

After a few meetings, the teacher received permission from the children for the practice teacher, Mr. Egely, to sit in. Ms. Brown asked the practice teacher to document how many times each child talked during the group *and* to whom the comments were directed. After the meeting, the two adults reviewed the information and realized that all of the comments made by the children were directed to Ms. Brown. The lead teacher spoke practically half of the time during the session. Ms. Brown adjusted her methods of leading the group and encouraging children to talk. Soon thereafter, children were talking more to each other, volunteering to share information, and expressing greater ease with what the group was accomplishing.

In summary, formative evaluation offers the practitioner access to information about events in such a way that review of activities can occur with relative ease. Information generated from the process can be instructive to the professional or colleagues because it provides details on the flow of events as well as on the interactions that were relevant to insuring that activities were carried out. When things don't go smoothly and produce the outcomes that the practitioner desired, the professional can review notes on agreements and activities to discover if something was missing from implementation plans (see Box 7.2).

The practitioner maintains primary responsibility for all aspects of formative evaluation. No other professional or paraprofessional in

BOX 7.2. Sample Practitioner Record-Keeping Form

Child's name: ―――――――――――――――――――

Contact dates: ―――――――――――――――――――

Presenting problem:

Goals and priorities:
   1.
   2.
   3.

Target dates for completion:
   1.
   2.
   3.

Statement of contract with student:

Contact with parents?

Contact with school staff?

Contact dates and topics discussed:
   1.

   2.

   3.

   4.

   5.

Evaluation:
   Verify completion of planned activities
      1.
      2.
      3.
   Verify projected outcomes
      1.
      2.
      3.

Follow-up plans:

the school system will be in a better position to insure that reliable and valid information is gathered on counseling process. Because of the fact that the professional cannot rely on colleagues to collaborate during formative evaluation, the school practitioner must decide on the content as well as structure of all components of this segment of evaluation.

Formative activities need not begin from scratch. Many school districts have begun to require that individual practitioners document to varying degrees the range and intensity of their professional activities. For example, people who are involved in counseling might have to provide a semester or yearly report that indicates how many students were involved, the length of time that involvement lasted on average, or other facts considered relevant by administrators. As might be expected, such documentation has limited value to the practitioner and serves instead to enter some report that administrators will submit. On the other hand, the types of information that administrators consider important can coincide with what the practitioner considers part of formative evaluation. Any reports provided in connection with the formative evaluation effort can be used as a supplement to requests from administrators for documentation. However such reports are used, professional school practitioners owe it to themselves and their colleagues to insure that their efforts are recorded for future review and reflection.

LOOKING AT PRODUCTS OF COUNSELING

When evaluation is included in most counseling efforts, emphasis tends to be on outcomes or products. Summative evaluation has a surface validity that can motivate practitioners to report outcomes. Administrators, as mentioned previously, are very interested in just this aspect of a total program of service.

Blocher (1966) has provided professionals with some criteria by which outcomes for clients can be assessed (Box 7.3). The four types include social adjustment criteria, personality criteria, vocational adjustment criteria, and educational criteria. Each set of criteria relates to the options available in the creation of counseling activities.

Social adjustment criteria look at how the child has changed in terms of interactions with parents, teachers, and siblings. Adjustments can be documented in terms of increases of positive behaviors, such as talking with parents, increases in participation in group activities (for example, choosing to work with peers rather than solo), or reductions in previous problem behaviors (for example, referrals for

BOX 7.3. Evaluating the Products of Counseling

Blocher (1966) suggests considering:

1. Social adjustment: how the child has changed in terms of interactions with parents, teachers, and peers.
2. Personality: how the child's self-esteem, locus of control, or related personality construct has changed (according to available assessment information).
3. Vocational adjustment: how the student has become involved in activities to develop specific vocational plans and how he/she has implemented such plans.
4. Educational performance: changes in academic outcomes (grades) and behaviors that support productivity (on-task behaviors, homework, etc.).

Feedback from students, school staff, and parents can be used to supplement information gathered by direct observation, record keeping, and the review of products (for example, assignments completed).

---

discipline). Adjustment issues often are the motivating factor that led the client to counseling. Whether the student, parent, or teacher initiated service, criteria can be selected to reflect the priority of service, specifically the goals and objectives for changes.

Theoretical orientation of the professional as well as the focus of efforts (individual versus group) will play a role in what is considered important in terms of changes. An Adlerian practitioner, for example, will place a high priority on a student becoming involved in family activities and taking greater responsibility for his/her own behaviors. A behavioral-oriented person, in contrast, will have already documented baseline information on the student's behavior and then, when counseling is completed, have a ready point of reference to take note of changes that have occurred.

Personality criteria as a category are a little more difficult to implement and interpret. Looking for changes in the way a client or a teacher describes the student along dimensions of a personality instrument is limited information at best compared to the more concrete descriptions available under the social adjustment category. A common activity in this category includes having the student complete an instrument of self-esteem or locus of control or a related personality inventory. Such measures, although widely used, were not intended by publishers to be used as test–retest tools to document change. With limited reliability and validity, these instruments contain such a wide margin for error that changes in the student's perceptions or behaviors will be masked within the broad true score range. The lower the reliability of an instrument, the wider the room for error in measuring any aspect of thought or behavior.

Vocational adjustment criteria are widely used when counseling activities relate to issues of career and work performance. Students who are unsure about their future plans for a vocation can turn to the practitioner for guidance and assistance. The adult can assist by involving students in activities to develop specific vocational plans and can advise students on applications for jobs, employment, or advancement on the job. Activities under this option can involve documentation of specific behaviors or activities of the student and thus are relatively easy to assess. In addition, the professional can seek reports from a client or professionals at the work site on such dimensions as the student's performance, satisfaction of supervisors, and the student's relative comfort with work responsibilities.

Career and vocational education programs contain within them vocational interest and aptitude measures that have been used to assess changes in students' thoughts and actions. Instruments available in the vocational criteria area are not intended by most educational publishers to serve as pretest–posttest measures to reflect student change. The practitioner is urged to review manuals or instructions provided with vocational instruments to be sure that an individual assessment tool is being used according to proper standards.

The final category to assess students is also a common one, that of assessing changes in students' educational performance. Products included under the educational criteria may be changes in grade point average and changes in academic behaviors that support productivity (measures of homework, classroom participation, and completing supplementary activities). In addition, George and Cristiani (1986) report the use of measures under this category that reflect school attendance and school participation. The practitioner can maintain records of truancy, tardiness, and dropout rates in an attempt to see if changes occur at the level of an individual client, groups of clients, or whole school programs. When changes occur within the area of educational variables, parents, administrators, and students have a clear sense that progress has been made.

In addition to investigating these four criteria areas or products, many school practitioners also request specific feedback from students on the completion of activities. Occasionally, such feedback is solicited on an anonymous basis. All students who receive services in a given semester can be sent a form asking them to rate what they liked or didn't like about the activities they experienced. Other professionals ask each student to fill out a form that provides information about what seemed to work and what didn't. Direct solicitation of feedback can intimidate some students but does offer the professional the opportunity to direct the students' attention to items of interest and to emphasize the importance that the practitioner is attaching to the feedback.

Another option available is to solicit feedback from the parents, teachers, or administrators who initiated the counseling referral. Have those adults who work with the student on an ongoing basis noticed some changes? Have they been satisfied with those changes? What give and take has been built into activities with the client to incorporate major concerns and priorities of the referring adult? Many such questions can be addressed in a follow-up questionnaire or form sent to the relevant adults in the child's life.

A more elaborate approach to generating information on what has occurred during the course of counseling is one suggested by Bergan (1977). In writing about behavioral consultation and counseling, Bergan has suggested that an interview can be used with the client or the referring adult to evaluate the effectiveness of the plan, revise the plan if a goal has not been attained, discuss procedures for maintaining behavior change, and return to an earlier phase of the counseling effort if new problems are introduced.

In one situation, a counselor requested that the client and the parent appear to discuss what had occurred during the course of a program of counseling. In this situation, the seventh grade student, Janine, and her mother came to the counselor's office after the completion of a 7-week series of counseling activities. All activities involved individual counseling with Mr. Simpson, the only school counselor. Mr. Simpson led off the meeting by asking the mother, a single parent, for her impression of how things had been going since their initial contact. By way of reference, Janine had come to the counselor with the mother at the encouragement of the homeroom teacher. Janine had been in many difficulties with other teachers in the school, was having difficulties with peers, and had had several run-ins with the mother. A common theme across all these had to do with the choices Janine was making and initiating in her actions. Janine consistently was being critical and what the mother labeled rude to others, using her actions to get attention.

Janine realized that her words and actions were offending others but was choosing to maintain her actions. The mother approached the school somewhat reluctantly and told the counselor her hesitancy stemmed from her own experiences in growing up. Mr. Simpson was able to develop a level of trust with the mother and child so that both agreed to a plan that would involve Janine in meeting with the counselor to learn and practice strategies of initiating and maintaining effective communication.

Janine's mother had indicated over the telephone to Mr. Simpson that she was impressed not only by Janine's behavior at home but by what she called her attitude. Janine seemed happier according to the mother and more tolerant of situations in which she previously would have expressed frustration at home. The counselor asked the mother if Janine needed any more time to work on some of the activities that had been begun with the counselor and the homework assignments that had been provided to her to insure she tried out certain activities. The mother consistently indicated her perception of success of the counseling. Janine echoed this evaluation and made some promises to continue working hard to be less offensive to others. The counselor then shifted attention to what could be done to be sure that Janine maintained some of the gains that had occurred. Included in this portion of the meeting was a discussion about how Janine's new behavior was affecting mother–daughter interactions. Both were comfortable and happy about the changes that were occurring and wanted to be sure they continued. To insure that, Mr. Simpson suggested a weekly meeting between the mother and daughter to review what had gone on during the course of the past 7 days. This meeting would allow both to air some differences and to see if future adjustments had to be made to how the two interacted.

Mr. Simpson promised to remain a resource to both and to be on hand if some negotiation was necessary. Janine and the mother were both satisfied with this agreement and promised to maintain contact with the counselor on at least a monthly basis.

School practitioners are well aware of the importance of maintaining a bridge between themselves and clients and family members. Open lines of communication will increase the likelihood that new problems are brought to the attention of the professional. An additional issue is of importance, however, and coincides with the professional's concern for the future of the student. Some students have problems generalizing what they learned in counseling activities to new settings and to new situations or may have difficulty maintaining levels of performance when not under the direct supervision of the professional. The vast literature on training students to generalize, developed by investigators working with handicapped children, has pointed out that if you expect the child to generalize behaviors to new situations you must train that child to do so. Thus, one of Mr. Simpson's activities with Janine later in the course of his involvement was to have her practice her new approach to communication with an increasingly wide range of peers and adults in the school, at home, and in the community. By giving Janine homework assignments to attempt such actions, Mr. Simpson was hoping that Janine would experience more and more success with her changed behavior. As it happened, Janine was quite successful in setting off on a new course of talking with others. If she had not been successful, Mr. Simpson would have had valuable information on her difficulties and could have made adjustments during direct contact to begin a greater emphasis on role playing or modeling of behaviors or could introduce her to a more intensive form of social skills training.

Being sure that gains and behavior are maintained relates to the development of the child's skill to generalize behaviors to new settings. Maintenance, however, involves not only the interests and actions of the client and professional but also important others in that child's environment. As a result, the adults in the child's life, whether at school or at home, can be alerted to what the child is now able to do so that recognition of changes and support for ongoing efforts to behave in new ways can be part of classroom and family life.

Bergan (1977) provides more detail for those professionals interested in evaluating changes in behaviors linked to the counseling effort. He discusses the option of evaluating programs that are preventive in nature versus those that are remedial or, as he calls them, problem centered.

A developmental interview and a problem-centered interview share in common certain objectives to look at goal attainment, to provide consultation or guidance as a follow-up to service, to reflect on plan effectiveness, to begin planning for most counseling experiences, and to establish procedures for follow-up activities (Box 7.4). The developmental interview will involve a number of key components under each objective. Goal attainment will involve an evaluation of the objectives that were established for changes in the client's performance. Did expectations initiated early on in a program aimed at prevention match the eventual outcomes for the child or children? Both primary and subordinate objectives can be assessed in a general way, as can the much broader goals for the total program.

Meeting to evaluate a preventive program can involve recognition that goals for prevention and the activities based on those goals were not meeting the needs of the clients or practitioner. Returning to an earlier phase of activities, even revising original goals and objectives, will fall within this component of the developmental interview. When the practitioner and client agree that activities have been implemented appropriately and as planned, activities can shift to the next component.

Plan effectiveness is a set of procedures that can resolve key questions bearing on the products of the developmental or preventive program. Bergan suggests that the professional examine sources

BOX 7.4. Evaluation Issues—1

Bergan's (1977) developmental interview
Evaluate goal attainment
Evaluate performance objectives and subordinate objectives.

Consultation/guidance
Determine if there is a need to return to an earlier stage of counseling (for example, reconsider priorities).

Plan effectiveness
Consider whether changes might have resulted from other influences than the planned intervention.
Assess whether the planned activities have resulted in real (observable or reported) differences in the student's life.
Evaluate whether new behaviors are generalizing to other settings than those initially targeted.

Postimplementation planning
Determine follow-up contacts and strategies as needed or as agreed.
Decide how to deal with new problems or concerns as they arise.

Procedure
Schedule future contacts or complete termination.

from within and external to the counseling arrangements that could have negatively affected overall effectiveness of the plan. If, for example, activities were not implemented on time or led to conflicts between participants in a group activity, evaluation of the products of counseling might reflect less the strength of the activities and tactics than the behaviors that interfered with total implementation priorities. Similarly, if events external to counseling tended to limit the scope or products of the counseling efforts, the school practitioner could establish the sources of such influence and then evaluate, if at all possible, the extent to which these were factors in eventual outcomes. For example, if a group counseling activity program was planned during the latter part of the school year and several sections had to be canceled because of class activities, the practitioner, in all fairness, should attempt to assess the quality of the original goals and objectives, the plans that went into creating a program, and balance this against the problems created by having students meet for what was intended to be a minimal number of sessions. Clearly, the professional should not establish a standard for excellence or perfection that ignores the influence of internal and external sources of invalidity. Bergan suggests that even in the most trying of circumstances, the professional can maintain records and evaluations of what has occurred and build on successes and mistakes when creating future interventions.

When assessment of products and process has been completed, Bergan suggests that the professional work with the client to establish strategies and tactics as a follow-up to prior activities. Bergan encourages having the client record information about postcounseling actions and consequences. When problems occur, the professional and client may have established a procedure by which to handle such difficulties so that the client feels more confident in returning for service. If such a link has not been discussed or established, the client may be very hesitant to "bother" the professional.

A problem-centered interview will share many of the characteristics of a more developmental one (Box 7.5). During goal attainment, evaluation of the behavioral goals will occur. Because Bergan has developed a plan that adheres significantly to the behavioral philosophy, evaluation of goals involves collecting data on changes that have occurred in clients' frequency, latency, or duration of behavior and comparing those to information from baseline or preintervention stages. In addition, Bergan encourages professionals at the beginning or identification stage of involvement to project what they would like to see occur in terms of client behavior change. By projecting a standard for behavior, the professional has a level against which to evaluate the effectiveness of the specific plan.

As with the developmental interview, problem-centered efforts can involve returning, based on feedback, to earlier phases of counseling. When process and product issues are assessed, the professional can focus on issues of plan effectiveness. Internal and external sources that affected the plan can be considered.

Finally, working with the client to establish strategies, record-

---

BOX 7.5. Evaluation Issues—2

Bergan's (1977) problem-centered interview
  Differs in structure from the evaluation interview in one key area—goal attainment. Focus is on evaluation of the specific behavioral goals determined during problem identification and analysis.

  Other procedures (consultation/guidance, plan effectiveness, postimplementation planning, and procedure) follow similar actions.

  The developmental interview differs from the problem-centered option by (1) being concerned with changes in behavior that require relatively long periods of time to attain; (2) involving attainment of one or more long-term objectives; and (3) generally involving mastery of subordinate objectives (for example, prerequisite skills) related to long-range goals.

keeping procedures, and procedures for handling additional problems will lead to a termination phase of the counseling activities.

George and Cristiani (1986) note that in evaluating efforts, practitioners should not generalize what has been established to other professional practices or procedures. They note that there is a big difference between evaluation, in which an effort is made to deal with issues in a general fashion, and research, which allows greater rigor and control during data-gathering activities. A difficulty in all counseling, of course, is operationalizing events and products associated with activities so that experimental rigor can be achieved.

The authors similarly note another difficulty in drawing conclusions about treatment effectiveness. The difficulty centers around what can be labeled contamination of effects. Students involved in counseling activities, whether group or individual, are also subject to educational or training activities that can produce changes in their thoughts, words, or actions. Peers can provide an influence in modifying the way a student behaves. A difficulty in making interpretations based on an evaluation of efforts is that there is always room to question the potential generalizability of what has been discovered. At best, evaluation tells the professional that something has occurred and that some changes were a consequence of those activities. At worst, evaluation can show that something has not occurred as planned or that no perceptible changes have occurred in the client. A key component of evaluation is the satisfaction of the professional with what has been accomplished. In research, in contrast, the investigator must satisfy not only internal standards but also standards of other researchers. Evaluation results, by definition, will have limited application beyond the local circumstances and people who work within the service environment.

Given the limits of evaluation, should professionals devote time and energy to gathering evaluation information? The answer is a resounding *yes!* Without any attempt at evaluation, practitioners have little idea about how to sequence activities with clients, which materials appear to work best given certain problems, and what has occurred in terms of the progress and participation of the students across the duration of activities. If more rigorous control is desired to address questions surrounding a specific theory or model of techniques, the professional can be involved in a research program.

RESEARCH AND COUNSELING OUTCOMES

In trying to discover research that bears on counseling practices, the reader will find that only a few investigations have been attempted looking at the efficacy of specific procedures under controlled conditions. Rather, many of the studies available in the literature are surveys of professionals that involve comparisons of various approaches to service. Early studies have documented that there are indeed differences in counseling practices that relate to the theoretical or philosophical orientations of professionals. But do the different approaches or models have a bearing on the outcomes that can occur? This important question has not been answered. Instead, writers such as Reynolds, Gutkin, Elliott, and Witt (1984) have concluded that little evidence is available to suggest that a strategy such as counseling can be more effective than a program of service, such as behavior management, that focuses on producing specific changes that can be documented.

Studies that have been done on the effectiveness of individual approaches (Rogerian, Adlerian, rational emotive, etc.) have produced a smattering of evidence that these models can produce client changes. A difficulty that is common to many counseling approaches is that of definition of the input, process, and outcome variables. As mentioned earlier, an investigation of a child's self-esteem is off to a shaky start because of the difficulty of defining exactly what is meant by self-esteem. Even if a definition can be established by a professional interested in investigating self-esteem, the difficulty remains of how to assess that construct. Again, even if a measure is selected, characteristics of that measure, such as reliability and validity, are such that changes that result over the course of counseling sessions may be attributed more to regression to the mean than to actual changes in self-esteem.

George and Cristiani (1986) talk about the limited attempts that have been made in the counseling literature to deal with practitioner variables, client variables, and situational variables. Prior research has looked at issues such as the practitioner's age, gender, background and training, theoretical orientation, and role within the institution. Client variables have included similar dimensions as well as nature of the presenting problem and expectations for the counseling endeavor. Situational variables include nature of referral, agency within which the counseling occurs, and administrative priorities for service. The approach to looking at these levels of influence is not unique to counseling. Much of the recent consultation literature, an alternative strategy to counseling, has focused on a similar breakdown of factors with equivalent results. In other words, little that can guide the practitioner or influence decisions about practice has emerged from research dealing with practitioner, client, or situational factors. A broader set of literature on the effectiveness of psychotherapy has been similarly discouraging. In general, if a conclusion can be reached, it would be that the behavioral orientations do a better job of producing and documenting changes. This not unexpected conclusion reflects the priority given by behavioral practitioners to operationalizing presenting problems, gathering data to establish a baseline, and implementing procedures that insure generating data that reflect changes in target behaviors. The professional interested in conducting a rigorous program of research on counseling is directed to the professional journals, which of late have reported several efforts to pursue evidence on counseling effectiveness.

ISSUES IN EVALUATING A PROGRAM OF COUNSELING

When a school determines that counseling services are needed, administration concerns may center on costs involved in providing services, the impact such services might have on students, the perceptions that parents would have of the options, and the broader notion of the acceptability of activities to the school board and general community. Entire programs can be evaluated on any or all of these points.

Options for services can stem from one or more possible directions. Professionals in the counseling field can find many examples across the United States and Canada of how to structure a counseling program to direct attention at certain needs in the school. An abundance of traditional programs exist that can serve as a model for a counseling and guidance department. In addition, a wealth of new programs specializing in such themes as suicide prevention, drug abuse, and pregnancy prevention are available both in the professional literature and in the educational marketplace. Identifying models and services is an activity that takes time but has an important payoff in giving the school or the counseling professionals within that environment an opportunity to select models and components that best match local needs.

As services are implemented, the issue of evaluating the entire scope of operations becomes relevant to both staff and administrators. School boards are well known for wanting yearly reports on what is being done across the school district. Superintendents recognize this concern of school boards and direct administrators to gather information that can be included in reports. Periodic or ongoing documentation of activities thus can be a part of any counseling program. Yet such documentation may have only a limited impact on the way that a program is conducted or evolves. If, for example, the school district is only concerned with the cost of operations and the number of students receiving services, such information can be gathered so that everyone in the system is pleased but result in little impact on the actual services to the students. If professionals and clients are to be affected by the content and process of counseling, evaluation of services must be more sophisticated than a simple recording of numbers.

An alternative for the school program is to focus on the progress being made in individual and group activities and to synthesize available information in a way that staff and consumers have a better sense of what has been attempted and accomplished. Tabulating activities and documenting changes are parts of such an evaluation. In addition, feedback can be solicited from parents, students, teachers, and other people affected by the programs so that adjustments can be incorporated into services (see Box 7.6). Program evaluation can prove useful in alerting professionals to gaps in service, directing attention at components of service that are not working as predicted, and pointing out difficulties in scheduling or implementation. Reflecting on what is involved in the process and products of all aspects of service can be a mind-boggling activity but will motivate participants to make adjustments, deletions, and additions that can improve staff satisfaction as well as client outcomes.

One component of looking at an evaluation of a total program is to maintain statistics on all expenses involved in delivering services. Cost effectiveness is of concern at many levels of the school district, and the counseling program can aid the effort of documentation by keeping

---

BOX 7.6. Program Evaluation Questions

What are the components and extent of counseling services?

What role does individual counseling play in the total service plan?

What is the cost, on a per-pupil basis, of services?

Are counseling services a priority for parents? Administrators? Staff? What methods can be used to determine the perceived priority?

What is the evidence of the impact of counseling services on the individual student, the faculty, the school?

How acceptable are counseling services to students, their families, and school staff? If services are recommended, with what frequency are they pursued, and with what consequences?

Does the community (read taxpayers and the School Board) support the provision of a range of counseling services?

Are community members satisfied with the programs that counseling services can provide?

---

track of contact hours and level of staff energy devoted to working with a client or family, and associating those with eventual outcomes. Professionals are aware that work with an individual client involves more intensity and time than working in group settings. Preventive activities often involve larger client groups than remedial ones. All forms of activities that are components of the total program can be assessed so that some evidence is available of the actual costs, whether in time or effort, associated with activities. Documentation of cost effectiveness is not initiated so that expensive activities are eliminated but rather so staff have a better idea of how they are devoting their time and how that time relates to specific client changes.

An additional dimension of evaluating counseling programs also can be considered: that of acceptability. Acceptability of services has been found to be related to the client's as well as parents' impression of how effective services have been. Simple measures of how the client and parents perceive what is going on, whether they see interventions as logically connected to the presenting problem, can be gathered quickly. Studies in school and medical settings have shown that by considering acceptability, staff members can adjust intervention programs to insure cooperation as well as followthrough from clients.

An additional component of program evaluation centers on needs assessment. The counseling program can, on a regular basis, gather information from the community, parents, administrators, and other staff members concerning what services are needed to meet the needs of students and the community. One district conducted a needs assessment every 3 years city wide. Responses from parents were addressed primarily at academic issues as well as the prevention of drug abuse and suicide. Programs for academics and the prevention of suicide and drug abuse were considered successful by district staff but did not receive much publicity. Administrators decided to use the local newspaper, which had an educational reporter, to highlight current programs and to solicit other forms of parental input. The school administration elected, in cooperation with counseling services, to initiate a parent volunteer program so that parents who were interested could play a supportive role in programs within individual schools. Parent volunteers were solicited to provide information on a career guidance program, participated in some educational support activities such as tutoring, and also played a role in a segment of the drug awareness program.

Needs assessments can additionally identify priorities for service that have not been considered. In the same district, one item that received limited attention in the schools but stood out in comments from staff was a demand for more homework for students. School staff had no district-wide policy concerning homework, although members of the faculty and administration were aware of research highlighting the importance of homework activities. A study committee was appointed by the superintendent and included participation from all elements of the teaching and support staff. The following school year the school district did publish a policy on homework. Faculty and support staff played a key role in shaping that policy and maintained their involvement in soliciting feedback when the policy was implemented.

Needs assessments do involve time and a real expense for mailing out forms and soliciting information from parents or students. The impact on services provided within a district can, however, be immense. Parents are often much more supportive and complimentary of what the school is attempting than staff would ever expect. Needs assessments function to raise the awareness of community members on just what is occurring in schools. A side effect is, of course, to reinforce the idea that the school is open to input from parents, students, and the general community. The combination of publicity and providing a channel for exchange of information is one that is tough to beat and enhances school–community relations.

Whatever direction school administrators, teachers, and other school practitioners take to assess the range and impact of services, the quality of services will be enhanced. Without feedback or involvement from consumers, counseling services and the professionals responsible for them have little opportunity to learn from what they are doing and to make adjustments in priorities and tactics. Evaluation at all levels of counseling, whether individual, group, or program-wide, can provide school practitioners with a sense of accomplishment balanced with a sense of humility. By realistically assessing the strength and weaknesses of all aspects of counseling services, school practitioners will be better able to cope with present as well as projected needs of students, parents, teachers, and administrators.

8

Ethical and Legal Issues

In this chapter, the reader is presented with four situations that illustrate possible dilemmas that may face educators who choose to become involved with students and parents by offering the service of counseling. Next, we discuss what can be learned from professional codes of ethics, which can serve to guide professionals who become involved in counseling. A brief discussion of legal issues that have implications for those offering counseling is also included. Finally, certain strategies are suggested to help guide educators toward ethical and legally appropriate behavior.

ETHICAL DILEMMAS

Situation 1. Ms. Strayer was a school psychologist assigned to two schools in a medium-sized school district. Over the years, Ms. Strayer had become well acquainted with the Ford family.

At a conference with Mrs. Ford about the educational program for Shirley Ford, a 15-year-old ninth grader, Ms. Strayer and Mrs. Ford agreed to meet again at the home of the psychologist. At this meeting, Mrs. Ford disclosed some apprehension that her husband was striking Shirley. Although there had been no obvious signs of abuse, Mrs. Ford had found Shirley crying in her room on more than one occasion when she returned home. Ms. Strayer reassured Mrs. Ford and encouraged her to feel free to talk further about events at home. The two scheduled another evening meeting.

Situation 2. At a group meeting of tenth grade underachievers, one of the members disclosed that he and some friends frequently stole food items after school from a nearby convenience store. Mr. Hughes, the assistant principal leading the discussion, didn't say anything as the other group members razzed the student and began to swap stories about their experiences at shoplifting minor items of food, gum, and cigarettes.

Situation 3. Ms. Jenkins, an eighth grade science teacher, had been meeting with Jerry, a slow student in her class, for most of the school year. One afternoon, after listening to Jerry relate a particularly brutal exchange between him and his father, the teacher offered to let Jerry come home with her to spend the night with her husband and her family.

Situation 4. During a meeting after school to make up some homework, Rhonda told her fifth grade teacher that a high school student named Sal was out in the playground. Rhonda said that for 50 cents Sal gave "kids some really neat drugs, just like the ones they take up at the high school." Ms. Johnson, the fifth grade teacher, told Rhonda to stop looking out the window and to get back to work.

These four situations illustrate some of the varied issues that educators may be drawn into—from listening to cases of suspected abuse to learning about a crime committed by a student to wanting to help a student by "rescuing" the student from a particularly brutal situation. The choices faced by such educators as these also highlight ethical issues such as the duties of a mandatory reporter of abuse in situation 1, the legal obligations of an educator providing counseling to report a crime as in situations 2 and 4, and the rights of parents in situation 3. It is necessary for educators to be acquainted with relevant professional codes of ethics.

CODES OF ETHICS

The development of professional codes of ethics is usually done by a group or a committee composed of members of a professional organization. The intent of professional codes of ethics is a subject of some conjecture.

Some would assert that codes of ethics serve to protect clients, or the public, from harmful activities and that the intent of such codes is to protect society. It has been stated that professional codes exist to "protect the profession from governmental interference," "prevent internal disagreement and bickering within the profession," and "protect the practitioner in cases of malpractice" (Corey, Corey, & Callahan, 1988, p. 140).

Regardless of the many reasons for their existence, codes of ethics offer some guidelines and raise some issues relevant to those who may be offering or about to offer direct services to students. Relevant considerations include the welfare of students, the competency of the educator, the right to informed consent, the right to expect confidentiality, responsibility to terminate a relationship, and the suggested practice of consulting with a knowledgeable colleague (Box 8.1).

Student Welfare

Students have the right to expect that educators have their best interests at heart. The process of counseling, as has been seen, is a very personal one that may include a great deal of personal content. The staff member who becomes involved with a student to the extent of offering counseling is usually motivated by a desire to help the student. The staff member maintains this focus as the relationship develops. The welfare of the student, including avoiding doing harm to the student, is an underlying concern of the service provider.

Before considering other issues raised by codes of ethics, let's return to situation 1. Shirley Ford was the one whose welfare Ms. Strayer needed to focus on, even though she was an acquaintance of

BOX 8.1. Ethical Areas of Concern

Student welfare
    Students and their families have a right to expect that educators have their best interests at heart and that counseling will help the student.

Competence
    Students and families have a right to services from competent professionals. Codes of ethics specify competency at two points—entry into a profession and at all points during a school practitioner's career. The practitioner who counsels will adhere to a standard of competence as specified by professional ethics.

Informed consent
    Ethical codes specify that the student be informed of all consequences of choosing to be involved in counseling. Voluntary participation is a critical ingredient for success.

Confidentiality
    School practitioners who become involved with counseling assume the responsibility of maintaining confidentiality. Exceptions are few, and may be specified in state or professional codes.

Progress
    Ethical codes specify that a client can expect to perceive progress related to involvement with the professional. If progress does not occur, the professional will refer the student to another practitioner.

Mrs. Ford. All states have regulations that mandate that certain officials report suspected cases of abuse. The state guidelines provide that the reporter does not have to "prove" there is actual abuse before providing information to designated authorities. The welfare of Shirley may dictate that Ms. Strayer do more than "reassure" Mrs. Ford.

One more comment. There are many cases in which a staff member sees a student who is in need of specialized attention and not getting it. There will be many reasons for the lack of services to some students, including lack of trust, busy schedules, waiting lists, and unavailability of staff. The most helpful act that will affect the welfare of such students is for the professional who has the trust of the needy student and the time to offer counseling.

Competence

School psychologists are guided by a code of ethics that forbids them from engaging in activities or providing services outside their area of expertise. It is the responsibility of all professionals to ascertain the limits of their competence. As has been suggested frequently in this text, educators who question their own ability to counsel a student need to identify and contact a trusted colleague who can consult with them during the counseling.

However, as a caring staff member begins to listen to a troubled student, there is a fine line between attempting to analyze a learning problem and becoming involved in personal matters. Therefore, we contend that professionals can continue to listen to and to help students explore their difficulties.

The ethical professional is also guided by codes of ethics that state that one must continue to increase competence and to obtain experiences that lead to increased skill and knowledge (Corey et al., 1988). The provision of counseling to selected students offers one way that educators can live up to this guideline.

In situation 2, Mr. Hughes "didn't say anything" as the students in the group treated shoplifting in a joking, teasing manner. Perhaps his decision could be attributed to Mr. Hughes's uncertainty as to what the appropriate action was. On the other hand, Mr. Hughes may have been acquainted with his local and state statutes, which usually indicate that there is no obligation to report misdemeanors when the information is obtained within a trusting relationship. However, the values and beliefs of a group leader, just as for any teacher, are relevant to the type of leadership provided to students. Will it seem that by his silence Mr. Hughes somehow condones shoplifting? Will Mr. Hughes demonstrate later that he was competent when he returns the group's attention to the earlier episode and uses it for educational purposes?

Informed Consent

With the increased importance of the consumer rights movement and with the increasing incidence of malpractice suits, the issue of informed consent has been receiving greater emphasis within ethical codes. Helping professionals are urged to provide students with the information needed to make an informed choice. Therefore, when a professional believes that listening to a student is turning into counseling, there is an obligation to alert the student to what is occurring and to offer a choice, such as counseling from the "appropriate" source. The professional can look for signals that the student is comfortable with the ongoing counseling or begins to appear uncomfortable, miss appointments, and communicate in other ways that there is a need to discuss what is happening.

Voluntariness is a crucial component in the process of informed consent (Corey et al., 1988). The student will have a choice about continuing in a counseling relationship. However, the issue of student welfare, which probably caused the educator to become involved initially, may mitigate against just stopping the helping process when the student can, indeed, be receiving much needed service.

Situation 3 featured a rather routine sounding session between an eighth grade science teacher and a slow student. However, a dilemma is raised when the teacher offered to take the student home with her for the night. Informed consent will provide students with choices and with small gradients of choice. It is better to view the process of informed consent as a gradual unfolding of choices by the student rather than as a specific hurdle to master. Asking a student to go home with the educator, no matter how justified, places responsibility on the student for a major decision. In this case, Ms. Jenkins could have offered to become more involved with Jerry.

"Jerry, what's going on sounds very brutal. Do you mind telling me more about how your father treats you?"

Assuming the student was willing to continue discussing the matter, the teacher could have helped Jerry consider what options were available to him. Going home with someone might not be the best choice. If Jerry had been made aware of several alternatives, he could have been given responsibility for making a decision with less far-reaching consequences. Since there is no mention of reporting an abusive situation, Ms. Jenkins may be violating a state code mandating reporting such occurrences.

Confidentiality

It is important that students be treated with respect and have their right to privacy maintained. The educator who becomes involved has a responsibility to keep confidences. Many educators already believe this to be an important value. However, we are all acquainted with cases in which a teacher regales those in the faculty lounge with, "Wait until you hear this one. You won't believe the stupid thing so-and-so said today in class."

It is important that after obtaining consent from the student to continue talking about a problem, and after focusing on the welfare of the student, the counselor doesn't invade the privacy of a student by gossip or inadvertent statements.

In situation 4, Ms. Johnson has a right to consider her student, Rhonda, and her own feelings about what she is to do with the information, hearsay though it is, that there is a pusher in the playground. However, as so often is the case, Ms. Johnson may consider the welfare of Rhonda and of other students as more important than Rhonda's feelings about privacy. Again, the values of the individual will affect each decision. Hearsay evidence is often not sufficient reason for invading the privacy of another.

Termination

Professional codes of ethics for counselors emphasize the responsibility of the professional to terminate counseling in cases where the student is not receiving benefit. This guideline is important for all educators.

Usually the student who involves a staff member in the process of counseling has special needs and presents extenuating circumstances that are out of the ordinary. Therefore, expecting quick change or sudden improvement is not realistic. However, the educator has the responsibility to monitor progress and to note when there is a lack of change. In such cases, it does not further the welfare of the student to continue. In fact, persisting in "counseling" that is clearly not helpful inhibits the welfare of the student, since no referral is sought.

Often in group counseling, certain students will demonstrate that they are not benefiting from membership in the group. Let's return to situation 2. If the same member who bragged about shoplifting plays the same role in other sessions, becoming the center of attention and getting the group off task, Mr. Hughes needs to protect the welfare of other members and to consider removing the one student. Otherwise, the entire group may make no progress.

Consulting

It is important that educators who are beginning to offer counseling to selected students identify a trusted colleague who is familiar with accepted practice. The educator can then further the welfare of the student by receiving advice and by checking out, with the colleague, how the current counseling is going. Consulting is not an invasion of the privacy of the student if the consultant/colleague keeps the confidence.

A recent case (Board of Professional Affairs, 1987) found in behalf of the actions of a school psychologist who had counseled a student who later tried to commit suicide. Part of the finding cited the fact that the school psychologist had obtained supervision for herself from a trusted colleague. The supervision was seen as a factor in the finding on behalf of the psychologist.

As an educator becomes more involved and more caught up in the concerns of a student, the need for an outside resource, one who has no particular ax or viewpoint, becomes greater. The helper can lose sight of other choices for students in the zeal to help.

LEGAL DIMENSIONS OF SERVICE

Schools, as work environments, are firmly embedded in local, state, and national communities. Each of these communities contains laws and regulations that influence performance. Codes of ethics, described above as standards by which a professional can determine and judge performance, represent a set of considerations often separate from the spirit and the letter of the law. In this section, we discuss some issues that influence the practice of counseling in schools and highlight legal ramifications of portions of that practice.

Professionals in schools are trained to deliver certain services. The actions of professionals may be defined overtly in job descriptions or covertly in terms of expectations that parents or others have of educators and support professionals. States across the nation have developed policies for practice and certification or licensure statutes that define and restrict service delivery. Although codes of ethics may coincide with such policies and statutes, they can differ.

Consumers of educational services, whether students or their parents, are, in theory, protected by the rules and regulations imposed on professionals by local, state, and federal policies and laws. Indeed, if an action by a professional did not function in the best interests of a child, few people would argue that such an action had any place in a school.

Given the standards that are imposed on professional practice, how can a parent contradict what a school argues is in the child's best interest? One method that can be taken by a parent to remedy present or past injustices affecting a child is to file a tort. According to Connors (1981), a tort is "any civil wrong, independent of contract, that leads to student injuries (physical, mental, or reputation) or reduces the 'value' of a pupil by failing to deliver a quality education" (p. 2). Connors argues that torts tend to fall into the areas of pupil injuries, defamation of character, and educational malpractice.

Three simple examples that could illustrate the application of these areas might be (1) a student falling off playground equipment, (2) a child being called a loser, in front of a class, by a teacher, and (3) a child graduating from high school and never having learned to read beyond the third grade level (and without participating in a special education program). Teachers involved in any of these examples could be sued by parents, claiming either intentional interference or negligence in the delivery of educational services.

Law suits against educators, although growing in number, do not often result in judgments against the teacher. Educators are considered by courts to have basic obligations that, if fulfilled, can serve as grounds for a defense in a tort case. The basic obligations of educators include adequate supervision of students, proper instruction, and maintenance of equipment (Connors, 1981). In the examples above, a teacher could argue that adequate supervision was provided to a child yet an injury still occurred, that a student had been reprimanded in front of peers and that the reprimand did not exceed the boundaries of either taste or school district standards for discipline, and that the student with poor reading scores had been instructed appropriately and guided toward remedial services, which had been rejected by the parent.

The key point to recognize here is that although parents have the right to contest actions of an educator or a school (their right to do so is protected in the United States), the educator or school has similar rights and obligations that guide professional practices to insure specific levels, qualitative and quantitative, of service. Now, let us consider the issue of an educator delivering a service considered to be counseling by the parent, student, or professional.

LEGAL ISSUES IN COUNSELING

We have dealt briefly with the distinction between a person engaging in counseling-related activities on a short-term basis (for example, a teacher helping a student discuss problems and work toward more effective coping) and the person with the job title of "counselor" delivering an array of services that include individual and group counseling. The actions of the latter are frequently regulated by district and state policies, whereas those of the former are not (Box 8.2). Some school districts have eliminated positions for counselors (using the rationale of cutting costs) and have placed the burden of counseling students onto teachers. Districts need not build expectations for such counseling into contracts; they simply expect teachers to "carry on" as effectively as possible in addressing the personal needs of their children. Other districts, with formal counseling services, expect teachers to include activities within their classrooms that center on counseling themes (for example, self-esteem training, social skills, drug awareness, and suicide prevention programs).

In-service training may be available to prepare teachers for individual and group interventions that have a counseling theme, yet even the best of workshops does little to insure that applications of concepts and techniques are consistent with training received. Indeed, a major failing and source of frustration with in-services is the lack of follow-up with teachers to insure fidelity of application and to monitor effectiveness.

BOX 8.2. Legal Dimensions to Counseling

Students
  Rights as defined by the Constitution and court cases
  Protection, under the law, from abusive adults
  Basic obligations of educators to provide adequate supervision, proper instruction, and maintenance of equipment

Parents
  Rights as defined by the Constitution and court cases
  Right to due process for their child and themselves
  Right to demand services mandated by the federal government
  Responsibility for care and guidance of student

School practitioner
  Responsibility to conduct actions defined by contract of school district
  Responsibilities for mandatory reporting of specific behaviors/events (for example, abuse)
  Rights as defined by the Constitution and court cases
  Right to due process
  Protection by some state legislatures for services delivered within defined duties

Teachers are in an unfortunate position when they have minimal preparation for counseling activities yet are expected to deliver specific services. Activities that may satisfy district standards seldom match the standards of the counseling profession. Teachers have little defense (other than to argue that they did as they were ordered) when parents consider legal action to prevent or remedy the impact of classroom-based counseling activities. As noted above, torts can be presented in those instances when the parent believes that school services have failed to deliver programming in the best interests of the child.

The broader issue of the ethics of teachers engaging in activities for which they are inadequately trained has not been addressed often by districts or teacher unions. In the absence of a teachers' code of ethics, the courts may have the final say in determining what services can and cannot be delivered by teachers in the course of their employment.

Responsibilities attached to the role of the counselor involve consideration of the needs of the community, policies and priorities of the local school board, integration of state mandates for service, and legal statutes that may apply. States may have mandatory reporting of certain behaviors (for example, reports of abuse, threats of suicide) and may allow for limited application of confidentiality with children. In one school district in the southeast, counselors were expected to attend to the problems of students well outside the boundaries of the school. With an absence of local resources, children brought their concerns to school counselors, who, over the years, had developed their own network of support. Counselors were asked to use their best judgment in determining how information provided by students was to be handled—who needed to know about the issues raised and how best to serve the student client.

In a midwestern rural district, counselors were defined by state standards as providing services that would remain confidential except in those instances specified by mandatory reporting laws. One counselor, Ms. Armstrong, was sued by the parents of a teenager killed in an accident off school grounds. The parents claimed that Ms. Armstrong knew that alcohol was going to be served at a party planned by students and that consumption of alcohol led directly to the accident that killed their son. The counselor had discussed, in a session with a student, an upcoming party that the student said would involve drinking. The decision of the counselor not to intervene to discover whether alcohol would be consumed centered on the counselor's perception that her discussions with the student were confidential, did not involve mandatory reporting circumstances, and involved actions outside of the purview of the school district. State regulations were introduced in court to confirm that Ms. Armstrong was acting within the limits of her role discription and expectations for confidentiality.

Although the counselor in the preceding case did escape the consequences of the suit brought by the parents, the case did raise serious discussion in the community about the role of counselors, the problems of alcohol abuse, and strategies for dealing with drinking and driving. The counselor reported, 2 years after the suit was concluded, that she remained unsure as to whether she had behaved in the best professional manner. Her doubts have influenced her actions—she now spends more time defining the limits of confidentiality with students and is more active in proactive programs addressing substance abuse.

Some professional counselors work without the protection of regulations defining the limits of confidentiality or the protections provided with assignment to a counseling position. In districts that have no defined service policies, the professional working within the limits of ethical standards (such as those provided by professional organizations in counseling or psychology) is provided with guidance on the limits of service delivery without being afforded protection from legal consequences attached to services. How does the professional cope? By pursuing clarification, in writing, of job expectations, by acting within the limits of professional ethics, and by seeking liability insurance, which is becoming more and more common as school practitioners recognize that professional life is heavily influenced by the legal realities existing within communities.

As counselors and educators recognize the impact of legal issues on service delivery, professional groups will begin to advocate for stronger protection of school practitioners. Regulation of professionals extends beyond states to national bodies. The American Psychological Association (APA) and the National Association of School Psychologists (NASP) have separately created guidelines for school psychological services, established recommendations for certification or licensure, and worked to implement standards for service in individual states. The APA and NASP recommendations may differ or conflict on specific points, yet both organizations have recognized the importance of defining scope of practice, provisions for the monitoring and evaluation of services, and strategies for advocating for the profession.

Psychologists in one midwestern state established their own supervisory mechanism to insure that services were being provided in an ethical and case-appropriate manner. The state professional organization supported the creation of a supervisory board to guarantee consumers that services were monitored to insure compliance with best practices.

Whether school practitioners rely on state or local mechanisms to define and monitor services or collaborate to influence or develop policies, the end result is the same: establishment of expectations for service and definition of consequences attached to provision of those services. Authors of major counseling texts have provided specific guidelines for practitioners that relate to the influence of legal realities on services.

Hansen, Stevic, and Warner (1982) emphasize that the professional has the legal responsibility to "inform clients what her or his skills are, perhaps indicating the extent of preparation, experience, and limitations" (p. 441). A contract is, essentially, being established between the practitioner and client, influencing expectations of both parties and providing momentum and direction to sessions. In schools, contracts need not be written, although some documentation of expectancies and goals can serve to remind participants of the priorities established earlier. The contract can serve additionally as documentation to parents and administrators of the counseling endeavor and be the springboard from which assessment of student change is determined.

Burgum and Anderson (1975) remind counselors that liability for their actions tends to revolve around three themes: the counselor has acted outside of the limits of personal expertise, the counselor defames the character of the client, or the counselor invades the privacy of the child through illegal search. Liability can involve either the commission or omission of certain acts. The courts have yet to provide a clear definition of liability in any of the three areas. The broader group of professionals providing mental health services similarly faces ambiguity of limits and consequences.

The courts have not removed existing confusion as to what constitutes privileged communication, an issue affecting actions of *all* counselors. George and Cristiani (1986), for example, discuss the implications of the Buckley–Pell Amendment of Public Law 93-380 on confidentiality practices of counselors, recommending that "counselors critically examine their own record-keeping practices, limit their use of technical language, diagnostic labels, and such, and maintain only information considered critical to the counseling situation (p. 294)."

Hansen et al. (1982) separate privileged communication into three clusters: "privileges protecting the individual client, such as those precluding any forced self-incrimination; privileges protecting systems within society, such as those related to jurors; and privileges that protect functions of importance to society, such as counselor–client communication" (p. 446). The authors point out that the application of privileged communication statutes is qualified, or influenced, by regulations and laws mandating reporting of specific actions (such as threats of suicide or harm of others).

In schools, the practices of counseling are influenced at times by the perceptions of the professional related to available time, priorities and preferences of the system, and reflection on how school-based services will be received by the family or the community. The type of service provided to the student in an affluent suburban school will often differ from that received by the student in an inner-city school. Differences need not always favor suburban locations, yet students in these schools may have the funds to supplement school services with private sector professionals.

What can school practitioners conclude about the legal dimensions of their role? Simply, professionals in all settings face an ever increasing influence of court and legislative mandates on their actions. It would be nice to think that parents would seek the support of the courts to reinforce the actions of educators and support professionals, but instead the involvement of the courts is viewed generally as at best an intrusion and at worst a disaster. Given the flood of students entering law schools, school practitioners can expect an even greater involvement of the courts in school-based practices. As noted above, professional organizations have often taken proactive stances in regard to role definition and expectations by publishing and advocating for standards of practice and supervision. The courts take a very different stance than do professionals on the merits of specific services. The courts look for legal precedents to justify actions, whereas professionals consider available research and clinical reports to guide actions.

How then does the individual practitioner or group of professionals determine actions that will allow for ethical delivery of services and satisfy the boundaries established by legislation and the courts for acceptable service? This is not an easy question to answer, but one that deserves a response that considers what can be done to prepare practitioners at the training as well as service levels.

STRATEGIES TO ENHANCE ETHICAL AND LEGAL DECISION MAKING

School practitioners who act only in response to personal preferences or an individual definition of what constitutes common sense will experience some difficulty if subjected to scrutiny on their adherence to legal and ethical standards. Common sense and personal preferences are a wonderful resource that can influence decision making, yet both would exist independent of formal training in education, counseling, and psychology. Preservice preparation centers on helping students to recognize the limitations of past experience in guiding actions. As Schon (1987) has argued convincingly, most professionals do acquire, during training, a mastery of skills in conjunction with a deepened sense of the mysteries (that is, jargon and constructs) of the individual profession. Schon (1983) provides an equally convincing argument on the limits of professional services (see Box 8.3). The failure of many interventions by professionals can be traced to a simplistic conception of the presenting problem and a reliance on strategies that are short term in impact (see Box 8.4).

Training school practitioners in counseling skills can thus recognize the complexity of any change endeavor and hone skills in problem setting, problem identification and analysis, application of interventions, and evaluation of services. In addition, attention should be applied at all levels of training and in all courses to consider the influence of ethical standards and regulations on the provision of services. Professionals must be prepared to structure decision making to account for a full array of influences relevant to individual cases. Much publicity has been given, of late, to the development of courses in business schools to deal with the ethics of practice. Similar courses

---

BOX 8.3. The Reflective Practitioner Contract

As described by Schon (1983, p. 302), a student would expect the following:

1. To join with the school practitioner in making sense of his/her own situation and, in doing so, gain a sense of increased involvement and action.
2. To exercise some control over the situation being experienced as a problem; the student would not be wholly dependent on information and action that the school practitioner can undertake.
3. To be able to test judgments against the competence of the practitioner (to feel free to engage in give and take on issues related to the goals of counseling); to enjoy the excitement of discovery of knowledge about oneself, one's actions, and the thoughts and actions of the professional.

Schon contrasts his contract with the more traditional components:

1. To place oneself in the professional's hands and, in doing so, gain a sense of security based on faith.
2. To have the comfort of being in good hands; to need only to comply with advice and all will be well.
3. To be pleased to be served by the best person available.

BOX 8.4. Change Assumptions for the Reflective Practitioner

Schon (1983, p. 300) specifies that the reflective practitioner works to enact the following assumptions:

1. The practitioner is assumed to know what to do in a given situation but not act as if he/she is the only one with relevant and important knowledge. The professional's uncertainties may be a source of learning to the client and the practitioner.
2. The practitioner seeks out connections in the student's thoughts and feelings. The client's respect for the professional's knowledge will emerge from discovery within the context of working together.
3. The practitioner experiences a sense of freedom and of real connection to the student as a consequence of no longer needing to maintain a professional facade (all-knowingness).

Schon contrasts the above with the stance of a typical expert:

1. The expert is presumed to know (and can claim such) even in the midst of uncertainty.
2. The expert keeps distance from the client and holds onto the expert role, conveying warmth and sympathy as a sweetener..
3. The expert looks for deference and status in the student's responses.

---

are common in medical and law schools and in programs for counselors and psychologists. Training in legal and ethical standards is promoted by the American Psychological Association, which emphasizes training in ethics within its organizational standards for accrediting programs in applied psychology. Attention to legal and ethical issues best resides as an infused component of all training rather than as an add-on course that considers issues in isolation from practices.

In the schools themselves, district and building administrators in charge of counselors can support application of services in concert with legal and ethical standards by remaining aware of current policies and decisions influencing practice. Awareness of new information can be passed on to staff affected by developments. Administrators can encourage, by in-service training and staff programs, the consideration of legal and ethical influences. Again, consistent attention to the importance of influences is to be preferred to irregular attention to legal and ethical issues. Too often, districts react to mandates that originate at state and federal levels rather than prepare staff to apply standards consistent with best professional practices.

Individual professionals and their organizations can take a stance of collaborating with local, state, and federal agencies to influence the development of policy and to testify in cases that involve the input of professional specialists. The school practitioner who does not have well-developed standards of ethical practice is ill prepared for changes in job expectations. Each school practitioner can integrate training experiences with knowledge of job sites to deliver services that adhere to an ethical code. As discussed above, ethical practices are not considered above the law but do create a basis on which to argue for the legitimacy of services.

Ethical considerations, attention to the legal ramifications of actions, and awareness of the acceptability of an intervention can be combined to influence school practices. The last factor, acceptability, has recently been found to be related to ratings of the effectiveness of interventions. That is, interventions considered acceptable by parents and children are more likely to be implemented and considered effective than are less acceptable alternatives.

Consider the case of Mr. Torgeson, a school psychologist at a junior high on the West Coast. Over the years of working with students, parents, and colleagues, Mr. Torgeson had established a comfortable set of procedures for contacting parents, contracting with students, and delivering services. By keeping aware of his professional organizations' (state and national) positions on ethics and legal issues, he considered himself ready to deal with almost every type of presenting problem. He was realistic, however, in recognizing that neither codes of ethics nor the courts dealt with *all* of the complicated issues occurring with junior high school students.

For example, a continuing problem in his school was pregnancy of girls in the eighth grade. For whatever reason, girls in the eighth grade were much more likely than seventh or ninth graders to become pregnant. Although the school district had policies on making accommodations for pregnant students, little attention was given to educating students on the consequences of sexual activities. Mr. Torgeson worked with other school staff and area resource people to develop ideas for school and community programs that would address teen-age sexuality and teen pregnancies. With his peers, he appeared before the school board and city council to argue for specific services. He asked his state professional group for assistance in identifying what other districts had done to deal with similar problems.

At all times, Mr. Torgeson remained aware of fiscal limits to delivering the services he and his colleagues were considering. An additional emphasis in his work was attention to the needs and preferences of the community. As an advocate for teens, Mr. Torgeson recognized that not every citizen shared the same urgency for developing services.

All school practitioners face a similar dilemma—a desire for action that can be complicated by the preferences of consumers and the priorities of administrators. How can one deal with such a dilemma? We believe that any action in defense of an ideal is better than remaining passive. Yet actions must reflect best practices in service delivery, an awareness of ethical and legal concerns, and coordination with the needs of consumers. Deciding what to do with a client requires consideration of local school district policies balanced with the training and experience of the professional practitioner.

APPENDIX A
Theoretical Influences on Counseling

In an effort to assist readers who may not be completely familiar with certain counseling theories referred to in the text, this is a summary of the key concepts of Rogerian, Adlerian, and behavioral counseling. The sections of this segment include all the information necessary to understand references to the theories in earlier chapters. The reader is directed as well to Appendix B, which contains suggestions for additional reading.

ROGERIAN THEORY

Carl Rogers (1951) described human beings as functioning in a perceptual or phenomenal field that is reality for them. From the earliest days of life and continuing across the life span, a self-identity emerges from the perceptual field. This identity is labeled self-concept by Rogers. The self-concept becomes the basis for personal functioning. Individuals strive to achieve self-enhancement or self-actualization.

The developing child is characterized as having the capacity to discern those experiences that will positively or negatively affect the self-actualizing process. A child will work to achieve positively valued experiences while avoiding, as much as possible, experiences that are negatively valued. The family plays an important role in creating the environment within which the child develops a self-concept. Snygg and Combs (1949) argue that four elements relating to family structure contribute to the emerging self-concept: experiences of adequacy, experiences of acceptance, experiences of identification, and expectations that emerge later in life as aspirations.

Rogers (1951) introduces the concept of positive regard, a need for all humans, as an influence on the child's eventual self-regard. Family members, through early experiences, play an important role in shaping self-regard.

As the self-concept develops, the individual will accept only those perceptions consistent with already existing self-perceptions. Social psychological research has supported Rogers's ideas on the potency of early experiences on later attributions of worth.

In counseling a person with a poor self-concept or problems with self-regard, the professional must provide a threat-free environment in which to initiate change. Key elements to effective counseling include (1) two persons in psychological contact, (2) an incongruent client (Rogers's term for the client with problems related to self-perceptions), (3) a congruent professional who will provide counseling, (4) a professional who experiences unconditional positive regard for the client, (5) a professional able to experience inner feelings and attitudes of the client (that is, empathy), and (6) a professional who communicates unconditional positive regard for the client as well as an understanding of that person's inner frame of reference. Rogers also would argue the importance of the professional sharing his/her reactions to what is happening in counseling with the client (Rogers, 1951). The sharing is motivated by the congruence of the counselor. This giving of honest reactions is a way of modeling congruence for the client.

Carkhuff (1969) did extensive work in the development of Rogerian counseling concepts and in the empirical study of these concepts. He has discussed stages of skills to use in the counseling situation: empathy, respect, concreteness, genuineness, confrontation, and immediacy. The helping process can be divided into two phases—the downward or inner phase and the upward or outward phase. Initially, the professional will assess the nature of the problem and the way in which the client sees himself/herself. The next phase will be spent working to determine the direction for problem solving. Empathy, respect, and concreteness contribute to increasing the client's understanding.

The client, over time, will achieve greater understanding of the dimensions of the problem at hand, steadily working with the professional toward problem identification and action. Movement toward a solution to the problem will be affected by the nature of the relationship between the two parties and the degree of self-understanding achieved by the client.

Carkhuff (1969) discusses counseling as emphasizing movement of the client toward action while he/she is being introduced to problem-solving options. To succeed in his/her role, the professional must be genuine in his/her actions, be able to facilitate confrontation, and be able to focus on the relationship to maximize communication. Carkhuff's term for the counselor's sharing his/her reactions with the client is immediacy, by which is meant the description of occurrences between client and counselor in the present or here and now.

As counseling progresses, the professional discloses more and more feelings and concerns, modeling openness for the client in the hope of producing a higher level of self-disclosure. Genuineness and authenticity of feelings will include sharing of both positive and negative feelings and thoughts. By the end of a counseling relationship, both parties, ideally, will be comfortable exploring all relevant thoughts and feelings.

Immediacy, dealing with thoughts and feelings as they are being experienced (not as they are remembered), adds an important dimension to counseling sessions. The professional will work to focus the client's energies on feelings as they surface.

Confrontation of the client may be one element that adds to client self-disclosure. The individual unsure about how to deal with problems may hesitate committing to a plan of action. The professional must be willing to confront the client's inaction, if only to clarify for the client the consequences of choosing no plan.

The final outcome of counseling will be that a problem area will be defined and a plan of action inaugurated. The professional maintains a consistent emphasis on positive regard and genuineness while nurturing the client toward change.

ADLERIAN PSYCHOLOGY

Alfred Adler, through his writings and the work of his followers, has made important contributions to the theory and practice of counseling (Corsini & Wedding, 1989). His writings suggest that human beings have inherent creativity and a concern for the welfare of others. Each individual is seen as operating within a perceptual field uniquely his/her own. The perceptual field is influenced by events and interactions so that development is affected by important forces such as the family.

The child, at a young age, is confronted with his/her inadequacies, some an outgrowth of simple immaturity and others influenced by being dependent on others. Feelings of inadequacy can grow as the child realizes that the larger world cares little about the individual. A sense of inferiority is not seen as strictly negative, however. The individual is motivated to move and grow or, as Adler labeled the process, strive for superiority.

The family offers an environment within which the child can feel valued and be provided with the opportunity to contribute to the family's welfare. The child begins to experience a sense of belonging in the group from an early age, a manifestation of social interest that generalizes to the broader society.

Adler argued that the child should be given the opportunity to be a partner in the family. This can be accomplished, in part, by allowing the child to assume responsibility in line with his/her abilities (for example, responsibility for chores and feeding). Children can be expected to assume greater and greater responsibility as they mature, further reinforcing the sense of belonging to the group. The same principle of nurturing belonging would occur in the classroom as well as the family.

Dreikurs and Grey (1968) discussed in depth the concepts of natural and logical consequences. Such consequences exist in the child's environment and serve as influences on the developing child's actions and beliefs about the world. Natural consequences are defined as the logical or immediate results of a child's behavior, not imposed on him/her by an adult, but "by the situation itself, by reality" (p. 65). A child who ventures outside during a shower can expect to become wet, a natural consequence of exposing oneself to rain.

Logical consequences, in contrast, are maintained and administered by persons having authority in a system. Logical consequences differ from punishment in that they are administered in a fashion that is related to the nature and severity of the transgression and used only when the child's actions violated rules that reflect the social order. The child who throws a tantrum when not allowed to have a cookie can be allowed to finish the tantrum, be ignored by the parents, and not receive the cookie. Furthermore, if tantrums are a continuing behavior, the parents might choose to remove the child to his/her room until the tantrum is over.

From the theoretical writings of Adler have come many proponents of counseling, especially with younger children and their parents. These practitioners emphasize the importance of encouragement, again for the dual purpose of dealing with the immediate demands of a situation and also providing the child with a clear message that the process of dealing with environmental demands is as important as the products and behaviors a child might generate. Encouragement contributes to the feeling of belonging in that the adult is recognizing the child throughout an interaction, not just at its end. Adler wrote that children must be valued and recognized for their efforts. Strengths and assets are to be emphasized, rather than the child's shortcomings. Children who do not experience a history of encouragement and caring do not meet their need for belonging. Many of the problems that educators see children experiencing in the classroom may be related to deficiencies in the sense of belonging from a young age. A child may feel he/she belongs only by misbehaving.

Dreikurs and Grey (1968) identified four goals of misbehavior seen in children's actions: attention getting, power, revenge, and feelings of inadequacy. By observing a child's actions, we can identify the goal of misbehavior and tailor our response so that the child can experience the consequences of maintaining a mistaken set of behaviors.

An important concept in a child's life in families is the family constellation. Adler emphasized the impact of birth order on children's development and explored the influences of family members on each other. He was interested in the interactions of nuclear as well as extended family members.

The child eventually develops a life-style that represents a merging of influences on the child, especially on the child's interpretations of experiences. Professionals who practice Adlerian counseling work on altering the life-style so that the child can gain insight into attitudes and behaviors that are nonproductive. Dreikurs outlined a four-step process to working with a child in counseling: establishing a relationship, understanding the child's life-style, disclosure of the life-style so the child understands, and reorientation, to allow the child to acquire new beliefs and skills related to belonging. The counselor who implements these steps would utilize the techniques of warmth, understanding, interpretation—a main method of disclosing the child's life-style—and empathy.

Adler introduced the notion of a fictitious goal to account for the child's belief about what it takes to succeed and belong when such beliefs do not coincide with the social interests of the group (whether family, the classroom, or broader society). Reorientation activities can be enhanced if the counselor acts as a model, assigns the child tasks (such as attempting new responsibilities) that introduce and reinforce specific behaviors, and provides multiple opportunities for practice (such as involving the student in role-playing experiences).

BEHAVIORAL INFLUENCES ON COUNSELING

Counselors who seek to help clients by implementing ideas from experimental laboratories have created a number of strategies to produce change in the context of counseling. The consensus of writers in the area is that all behaviors, the positive and the negative, are learned as a direct result of consequences from the environment. Such consequences can involve the responses of others, natural consequences (similar to the Adlerian notion), and lack of a response. Behavioral counselors would argue that if a behavior can be learned, it can be modified or eliminated. Thus, the goal of behavioral counseling will be to modify specific behaviors of the client. Setting specific and concrete goals simplifies the task of evaluation in behavioral counseling, one of its advantages over other types of counseling.

If a behavior is followed by a positive consequence, the behavior is strengthened and more likely to occur in the future. Behavior is acquired using a process called positive reinforcement. Two broad classes of positive reinforcers are said to exist: primary reinforcers (such as food, water, shelter) and secondary reinforcers (including social actions, such as smiles, touch, and so on). Secondary reinforcers are defined as any stimuli that have acquired reinforcing properties (that is, increase the likelihood of a behavior occurring).

Negative reinforcement (a separate concept from punishment) is the process of removing an aversive stimulus from the environment, thus increasing the likelihood of the repetition of the behavior that led to the termination of the aversive event. For example, a child who is misbehaving may note that a teacher stops yelling when the misbehavior stops. If the lack of yelling is reinforcing to the child, the misbehavior is likely to decrease.

Punishment is defined as either the withdrawal of a positive reinforcer or the presentation of an aversive stimulus. A child who is crying might have a toy taken away or be spanked as punishment. Contrary to the opinion of some educators, behavioral counselors do not advocate the indiscriminate use of punishment, preferring to provide positive consequences to behaviors whenever possible. Punishment might be used in those special situations when other tactics haven't worked or when an immediate response is needed quickly to eliminate a behavior. The young child crossing a dangerous street without permission might be spanked to emphasize the danger of the action.

Another important concept relevant to helping students acquire new behaviors is shaping. Shaping involves the acquisition of complex behaviors through successive approximations of the skills that make up the total behavior. For example, teaching a child to write with a pencil can involve the teacher reinforcing the child for increasingly sophisticated use of the pencil in the writing process.

Writers such as Bandura (1971) argue that children can acquire new behaviors through imitation of models. Children are quite observant of their surroundings and aware of when their actions do not match those of others. By imitation, students can acquire, without our guidance, new or refined versions of behavioral acts.

Extinction is a concept important to weakening and eliminating existing behaviors. Ignoring a behavior is a common strategy that can lead, after an initial increase in frequency as the student tries to get our attention, to the eventual removal of a behavior. The teacher, for example, who observes a child's attempts at attention getting (such as arm waving) can ignore the behavior until the child opts to get attention in an approved fashion.

If the practitioner is interested in shaping new behaviors that are resistant to extinction, an intermittent reinforcement schedule can be used. The concept of reinforcement schedule relates to the manner in which we deliver reinforcement to a child. We can reinforce an action every time it occurs or do so less frequently (at random intervals or on some schedule). Research shows that a behavior becomes more resistant to extinction if we have used an intermittent schedule in the process of building the new, positive behavior.

An additional influence on learning is the closeness in time in which we deliver reinforcers after a target behavior. Again, research shows that reinforcers work best when delivered close in time to the behavior that we would like to see strengthened.

Discrimination is an important concept in the learning process. As practitioners, we would want a student to apply new skills in response to cues from the environment and use such skills in an appropriate manner. In addition, we also want students to generalize skills to other environments, again when appropriate. We also can work with students so that they do not need a specific cue to perform a behavior but will instead respond to a class of signals. Imagine a child just learning to behave in a socially appropriate manner with peers. After training students in social skills, the professional would attempt to have the students engage in these skills in the classroom and on the playground, eventually responding only to signals from peers (rather than adults) that social contact is appropriate.

Many other concepts have been developed to account for the opportunities adults have to influence the actions of children, whether to increase, maintain, or decrease the occurrence of a behavior. Bergan (1977) provides valuable information on the choices available for behavioral interventions.

Goals during behavioral counseling will specify which behaviors a client will change. The techniques for behavioral counseling, whether in groups or individually, involve the use of the concepts just described, including arranging reinforcement and punishment events contingent on the actions of the client, shaping desired behaviors by administering reinforcement to gradually increasing standards of behavior, providing models for the client, and helping the client learn to make discriminations.

Advantages of behavioral counseling involve its goals and the ease of evaluation. The specification of goals, although a difficult task, enables the counselor and client to understand the purpose of counseling. In addition, when appropriate, behavioral counselors can communicate the purposes of their involvement with clients in a manner understandable to administrators and to parents. By establishing specific goals, both the counselor and, more importantly, the client can note the progress being made. Are we getting anywhere? Am I meeting my goals?

APPENDIX B
Further Readings

ROGERIAN COUNSELING

Carkhuff, R. R. (1971). Training as a preferred mode of treatment. *Journal of Counseling Psychology, 18,* 123–131.

Landreth, G. L. (1984). Encountering Carl Rogers: His views on facilitating groups. *Personnel and Guidance Journal, 62,* 323–325.

Rogers, C. (1951). *Client-centered therapy.* Boston: Houghton Mifflin.

Rogers, C. (1961). *On becoming a person.* Boston: Houghton Mifflin.

ADLERIAN COUNSELING

Dinkmeyer, D. C., & Muro, J. J. (1979). *Group counseling: Theory and practice* (2nd ed.). Itasca, IL: Peacock.

Dinkmeyer, D. C., Pew, W. L., & Dinkmeyer, D. C., Jr. (1979). *Adlerian counseling and psychotherapy.* Monterey, CA: Brooks/Cole.

BEHAVIORAL COUNSELING

Franks, C. M., & Wilson, G. T. (1973). *Behavior therapy: Theory and practice.* New York: Brunner/Mazel.

Rose, S. D. (1977). *Group therapy: A behavioral approach.* Englewood Cliffs, NJ: Prentice-Hall.

COGNITIVE BEHAVIORAL COUNSELING

Ellis, A. (1982). *Rational–emotive therapy and cognitive behavior therapy.* New York: Springer.

Shaffer, C. S., Sank, L. I., Shapiro, J., & Donovan, D. C. (1982). Cognitive behavior therapy follow-up: Maintenance of treatment effects at six months. *Journal of Group Psychotherapy, Psychodrama and Sociometry, 35,* 57–63.

SKILL DEVELOPMENT

Corey, G., Corey, M. S., Callahan, P. J., & Russell, J. M. (1982). *Group techniques.* Monterey, CA: Brooks/Cole.
Egan, G. (1975). *The skilled helper.* Monterey, CA: Brooks/Cole.
Gazda, G. M., Asbury, F. S., Balzer, F. J., Childers, W. C., & Walters, R. P. (1984). *Human relations development: A manual for educators* (3rd ed.). Newton, MA: Allyn and Bacon.
Ivey, A. E., & Gluckstern, N. B. (1976). *Basic influencing skills: Participant manual.* North Amherst, MA: Author.
Johnson, D. W. (1981). *Reaching out* (2nd ed.). Englewood Cliffs, NJ: Prentice-Hall.
Masson, R. L., & Jacobs, E. (1980). Group leadership: Practical points for beginners. *Personnel and Guidance Journal, 59,* 52–55.

CONSULTATION

Alpert, J. L., & Associates. (1982). *Psychological consultation in educational settings.* San Francisco: Jossey-Bass.
Brown, D., Pryzwansky, W. B., & Schulte, A. C. (1987). *Psychological consultation: Introduction to theory and practice.* Boston: Allyn and Bacon.
Conoley, J. C. (Ed.). (1981). *Consultation in schools: Theory, research, procedures.* New York: Academic Press.
Gallessich, J. (1982). *The profession and practice of consultation.* San Francisco: Jossey-Bass.
Parsons, R. D., & Meyers, J. (1984). *Developing consultation skills.* San Francisco: Jossey-Bass.

References

Algozzine, B., Ysseldyke, J., Christenson, S., & Thurlow, M. (1982). *Teachers' intervention choices for children exhibiting different behaviors in school.* Minneapolis: University of Minnesota, Institute for Research on Learning Disabilities.

American Association for Counseling and Development. (1988). Ethical standards (3rd rev.). *Journal of Counseling and Development, 67*(1), 4–8.

Bandura, A. (1971). *Social learning theory.* Morristown, NJ: General Learning Corp.

Benjamin, A. (1981). *The helping interview* (3rd ed.). Boston: Houghton Mifflin.

Bergan, J. R. (1977). *Behavioral consultation.* Columbus, OH: Charles E. Merrill.

Blocher, D. H. (1966). *Developmental counseling.* New York: Ronald Press.

Board of Professional Affairs. (1987). Casebook for providers of psychological services. *American Psychologist, 42,* 704–711.

Brown, D., Pryzwansky, W. B., & Schulte, A. C. (1987). *Psychological consultation: Introduction to theory and practice.* Boston: Allyn and Bacon.

Burgum, T., & Anderson, S. (1975). *The counselor and the law.* Washington, DC: American Personnel and Guidance Association Press.

Carkhuff, R. R. (1969). *Helping and human relations: A primer for lay and professional helpers* (Vols. I and II). New York: Holt, Rinehart & Winston.

Carkhuff, R. R. (1973). *The art of problem-solving.* Amherst, MA: Human Resource Development Press.

Colangelo, N., Dustin D., & Foxley, C. (1982). *The human relations experience: Exercises in multicultural nonsexist education.* Monterey, CA: Brooks/Cole.

Connors, E. T. (1981). *Educational tort liability and malpractice.* Bloomington, IN: Phi Delta Kappa.

Corey, G. (1981). *Theory and practice of group counseling* (2nd ed.). Monterey, CA: Brooks/Cole.

Corey, G., Corey, M. S., & Callahan, P. (1988). *Issues and ethics in the helping professions* (3rd ed.). Monterey, CA: Brooks/Cole.

Corsini, R. J. (1984). *Current psychotherapies* (3rd ed.). Itasca, IL: Peacock.

175

Corsini, R. J., & Wedding, D. (1989). *Current psychotherapies* (4th ed.). Itasca, IL: Peacock.

Dinkmeyer, D., & Carlson, J. (1973). *Consulting: Facilitating human potential and change processes.* Columbus, OH: Charles E. Merrill.

Dinkmeyer, D. C., Pew, W. L., & Dinkmeyer, D. C., Jr. (1979). *Adlerian counseling and psychotherapy.* Monterey, CA: Brooks/Cole.

Dreikurs, R., & Grey, L. (1968). *A new approach to discipline: Logical consequences.* New York: Hawthorn.

Dreikurs, R., & Soltz, V. (1964). *Children: The challenge.* Des Moines, IA: Meredith.

Duncan, J. A., & Gumaer, J. (Eds.). (1980). *Developmental groups for children.* Springfield, IL: Charles C. Thomas.

Dustin, D., & Blocher, D. H. (1984). Theories and models of consultation: Research status and future directions. In: R. W. Lent & S. D. Brown (Eds.), *Handbook of counseling psychology* (pp. 751–781). New York: John Wiley & Sons.

Dustin, D., & Curran, J. (1985). Genuineness and self-disclosure in the classroom. In: N. Colangelo, D. Dustin, & C. Foxley (Eds.), *Multicultural nonsexist education: A human relations approach* (2nd ed., pp. 48–55). Dubuque, IA: Kendall/Hunt.

Dustin, D., Ehly, S., & Curran, J. J. (1984). Are counselors too busy to consult? *Iowa Journal of Counseling, 3(2),* 15–17.

Egan, G. (1975). *The skilled helper: A model for systematic helping and interpersonal relating.* Monterey CA: Brooks/Cole.

Egan, G. (1976). *Interpersonal living: A skills/contract approach to human-relations training in groups.* Monterey, CA: Brooks/Cole.

Ehly, S., Dustin, D., & Bratton, B. (1983). Evaluation of a consultation training component. *Teaching of Psychology, 10,* 222–225.

Ehly, S., Dustin, D., & Forsyth, R. (1985). A comparison between counseling and consulting activities of school psychologists and school counselors. In: J. F. Cruz, L. S. Almeida, & O. F. Goncalves (Eds.), *Psychological interventions in education* (pp. 37–42). Porto, Portugal: Associacao Portuguesa de Licenciados em Psicologia.

Ellis, A. (1962). *Reason and emotion in psychotherapy.* New York: Lyle Stuart.

Ellis, A. (1973). *Humanistic psychotherapy: The rational–emotive approach.* New York: Julian Press.

Gallessich, J. (1982). *The profession and practice of consultation.* San Francisco: Jossey-Bass.

Gazda, G. M. (1973). *Human relations development: A manual for teachers.* Boston: Allyn and Bacon.

George, R. L., & Cristiani, T. S. (1986). *Theory, methods, and processes of counseling and psychotherapy* (2nd ed.). Englewood Cliffs, NJ: Prentice-Hall.

George, R. L., & Dustin, D. (1988). *Group counseling: Theory and practice.* Englewood Cliffs, NJ: Prentice-Hall.

Gordon, T. (1974). *T. E. T.: Teacher effectiveness training.* New York: McKay.

Hansen, J. C., Stevic, R. R., & Warner, R. W., Jr. (1982). *Counseling theory and process* (3rd ed.). Boston: Allyn and Bacon.

Havighurst, R. J. (1951). *Developmental tasks in education.* New York: Longmans.

Ivey, A. E. (1983). *Intentional interviewing and counseling.* Monterey, CA: Brooks/Cole.

Ivey, A. E., & Gluckstern, N. B. (1976). *Basic influencing skills: Participant manual.* North Amherst, MA: Microtraining Associates.

Johnson, D. W. (1986). *Reaching out—Interpersonal effectiveness and self-actualization* (3rd ed.). Englewood Cliffs, NJ: Prentice-Hall.

Krumboltz, J. (1966). Behavioral goals of counseling. *Journal of Counseling Psychology, 13,* 153–159.

Lieberman, M. A. (1980). Group methods. In: F. H. Kanfer & A. P. Goldstein (Eds.), *Helping people change* (2nd ed., pp. 470–536). New York: Pergamon.

Marlowe, R. H., Madsen C. H., Bowen, C. E., Reardon, R. C., & Logue, P. E. (1978). Severe classroom behavior problems: Teachers or counselors. *Journal of Applied Behavior Analysis, 11,* 53–66.

Maultsby, M. C., Jr. (1975). *Help yourself to happiness through rational self-counseling.* Boston: Marlborough House.

Neely, M. (1982). *Counseling and guidance practices with special education students.* Homewood, IL: Dorsey.

Prout, H. T., & Brown, D. T. (1983). *Counseling and psychotherapy with children and adolescents: Theory and practice for school and clinic settings.* Tampa, FL: Mariner.

Reynolds, C. R., Gutkin, T. B., Elliott, S. N., & Witt, J. C. (1984). *School psychology: Essentials of theory and practice.* New York: John Wiley & Sons.

Rogers, C. (1951). *Client-centered therapy.* Boston: Houghton Mifflin.

Rogers, C. (1972). Foreword. In: L. N. Solomon & B. Berzon (Eds.), *New perspectives in encounter groups* (pp. viii–xi). San Francisco: Jossey-Bass.

Schon, D. A. (1983). *The reflective practitioner.* New York: Basic Books.

Schon, D. A. (1987). *Educating the reflective practitioner.* San Francisco: Jossey-Bass.

Snygg, D., & Combs, A. W. (1949). *Individual behavior.* New York: Harper.

Stewart, N., Winborn, B., Johnson, R., Burks, H., & Engelkes, J. (1978). *Systematic counseling.* Englewood Cliffs, NJ: Prentice-Hall.

Stone, F. B. (1981). Behavior problems of elementary school children. *Journal of Abnormal Child Psychology, 9,* 407–418.

Stone, G. L. (1980). *A cognitive–behavioral approach to counseling psychology.* New York: Praeger.

Warner, R. W., Jr. (1980). *Individual counseling.* Atlanta: Georgia Department of Education.

Yalom, I. D. (1985). *Theory and practice of group psychotherapy* (3rd ed.). New York: Basic Books.

Index

Academic performance, 137
Acceptability of services, 147, 164
Acceptance, and rapport, 60, 61
Acting-out behavior, 36
Active listening, 124
Adlerian approach
  group counseling, 91, 92
  individual counseling, 82–84
  key concepts, 4–6, 13, 168–170
Adolescents, counseling problems, 31
Advice, 56
Aggressive students, 99
American Psychological Association, 159

B

Behavior change, 36
Behavior management, 12
Behavioral techniques
  advantages, 172
  baseline data, 79
  evaluation, 45
  group counseling, 93, 103
  individual counseling, 78–81
  key concepts, 6, 7, 13, 170–172
  outcome studies, 144, 145
  specificity, 79, 80
Boys, counseling problems, 31, 32
Buckley–Pell Amendment, 160

C

Clarification, 50
Client-centered therapy, 3, 4, 13, 166–168

Closed questions, 48, 49
Codes of ethics, 150–155
Coercion, 100
Cognitive behavioral counseling, 7–10, 13
Communication, and rapport, 60, 61
Competence, and ethics, 152, 153
Confidentiality
  and legal responsibility, 158–160
  and privileged communication, 160, 161
  and referrals, 16
Consultation
  versus counseling, 19–22
  ethical issues, 155
  problem definition, 20
  and referral issues, 15
Consultee, definition, 19
Contracts
  behavioral techniques, 80
  counseling interventions, 43
  and evaluation, 131
  legal issues, 160, 162
Coping skills, 36, 37
Cost effectiveness, 146
Counseling, definition, 1–3
Crisis intervention
  coping skills, 37
  individual counseling, 84

D

Decision making
  counseling effectiveness, 12
  counseling goals, 37, 38

Decision making (*continued*)
 and problem analysis, 71
Democratic structures, 83
Developmental interview, 140–142
Direct questions, 49
Direct services, 18, 19
Discrimination (learning), 171, 172

E

Educational performance, 137
Ellis's approach, 7–10, 13
Empathy
 and rapport, 61, 62
 Rogerian theory, 4
Encouragement concept, 82, 169
Ethical issues, 149–165
Evaluation, 129–148
 criteria, 135–137
 developmental interview, 140–142
 and feedback, 137, 138
 individual counseling, 43–45, 75–78,
  129–148
 problem-centered interview, 142, 143
Explanation, 54
Extinction, 171

F

Family constellation, 169
Family structure, 5
Feedback, 137, 138
Fictitious goal, 170
Follow-up, group counseling, 107
Formative evaluation, 44, 129–135
Friendliness, counseling skills, 26

G

Generalization of behavior, 139, 140
Genuineness
 counseling skills, 27
 Rogerian theory, 4
Girls, counseling problems, 31, 32
Goals
 behavioral counseling, 172
 and evaluation, 140
 individual counseling, 34–36
Group counseling, 88–128
 Adlerian approach, 91, 92
 behavioral approach, 93, 103

content issues, 123–128
follow-up, 107
goals, 89–98
and individual identity, 102
interpersonal learning in, 97
leadership techniques, 116–122
membership criteria, 95, 96, 100, 101
orientation stage, 102
process of, 109–116
Rogerian approach, 90, 91, 103
termination, 104, 105
Group membership criteria, 95, 96,
 100, 101

H

Handicapped students, 35
Heterogeneous groups, 100, 101
Homework, 43
Homogeneous groups, 100, 101
Hostility, 121
Humor, 26

I

Identification of problem, 39–42, 62
Imitation, 171
Indirect questions, 49
Indirect services, 18, 19
Individual counseling
 Adlerian approach, 82–84
 behavioral techniques, 78–81
 crisis intervention, 84
 evaluation, 43–45, 75–78
 evaluation form, 78
 goals, 34–36
 identification of problem, 39–42, 64–
  69
 implementation, 47, 48
 intervention stage, 43, 73–75
 outcome studies, 143–145
 proactive intervention, 84–86
 problem analysis, 42, 69–73
 problem setting, 62–64
 and rapport, 59–61
Individual identity, 102
Individual psychology groups, 6
Informed consent, 153
Insight, 90, 91
Intermittent reinforcement, 171
Interpersonal learning, 97

Interpersonal relationships
  counseling evaluation, 135, 136
  counseling goal, 38
Interviewing, 48–58
  open versus closed questions, 48
  problem analysis, 42
  skills, 48–58

L

Leads and responses, 59, 58
Legal issues, 149–165
Liability, 160
Life script, 91, 92
Life-style, 5, 170
Logical consequences, 82, 83, 169

M

Maintenance of gains, 140
Malpractice, 156
Maultsby's approach, 7–10
Minimal encouragers, 49
Minors, referral issues, 16, 17
Modeling
  behavioral theory, 171
  in group counseling, 97, 98
Moralizing, 57, 58
Motivation, 100

N

National Association of School Psychologists, 159
Natural consequences, 169
Needs assessment, 147, 148
Negative reinforcement, 170, 171
Nonverbal behavior, 61
Normalization, 35

O

Open questions, 48, 63, 125
Outcome studies, 143–145

P

Paraphrasing
  group counseling, 118, 125
  individual counseling, 50, 53, 63

Parental permission, 32, 33
Parents
  counseling evaluation, 138, 139
  informing of, 44
  legal rights, 157
Partner Observation Form, 28
Passive behavior, 31, 32
Peer relationships
  counseling goal, 38
  intervention, 75
Personal responsibility concept, 83, 84
Personality, 136
Positive reinforcement, 170, 171
Prevention programs
  evaluation, 140
  individual counseling, 45, 46, 84, 85
Primary reinforcers, 170
Proactive interventions, 84–86
Problem analysis, 42, 69–73
Problem-centered interview, 140, 142
Problem identification, 39–42, 62
Problem ownership concept, 83, 84
Problem setting, 62–64
Problem solving
  and problem analysis, 70, 71
  steps in, 40
Psychotherapy, versus counseling, 2
Public Law *93-380*, 160
Punishment, 171

Q

Questioning techniques, 48, 49, 124, 125

R

Rapport, 59–62
Rating scales, 132, 133
Rational behavioral therapy (Maultsby), 7
Rational emotive therapy (Ellis), 7–10, 13
Record keeping, 133, 134
Referral, 14–18, 45, 66, 67
Reflecting meaning, 63
Reflection of feelings, 4, 50–53
Reinforcement schedule, 171
Research, counseling outcome, 143–145
Resistance, 121
Response versus lead distinction, 49, 58

Restatement, 50, 117, 125
Rogerian approach
    group counseling, 90, 91, 103
    key concepts, 3, 4, 166–168

S

School attendance
    counseling evaluation criterion, 137
    individual counseling, 85
School boards, 145, 146
School participation, 137
Secondary reinforcement, 170
Self-acceptance, 12
Self-actualization, 166
Self-concept, 166–168
Self-control, 39
Self-disclosure
    counseling skills, 27
    group counseling leaders, 122,
        122
Self-efficacy, 12
Self-monitoring, 81
Self theory (Rogers), 3, 4, 166–168
Shaping, 171
Shyness
    girls, 31, 32
    group counseling, 99
Silence, 49, 121
Social adjustment, 135, 136
Social learning, 97, 99
Social skills
    counseling intervention, 75
    group counseling, 97, 127, 128
    individual counseling, 85
Social support, 97
Special education students, 35

Stress
    coping skills development, 36, 37
    group counseling, 97
Student rights, 157
Student welfare, and ethics, 151, 152
Study skills, 97
Suggestion, 55, 56
Summaries, group counseling, 125, 126
Summative evaluation, 44
Supervision, 15
System-wise skill, 29

T

Teachers
    consultation, 12
    legal issues, 156–158
Termination stage
    and ethics, 154
    group counseling, 104, 105
    individual counseling, 77
Time constraints, 24
Torts, 156
Truancy, 85
Trust
    counselor characteristics, 26
    in group counseling, 112
    and rapport, 60, 61

U

Unconditional positive regard, 4

V

Voluntariness, and informed consent,
    153